The Female Fat Solution

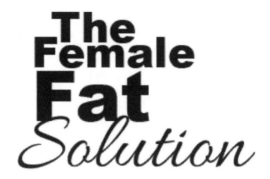

The Female Fat Solution

Achieving lasting
weight loss by getting
your hormones to work
for you!

Dr. Beth Westie

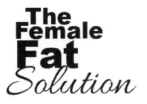

Achieving lasting
weight loss by getting
your hormones to work for you!

ISBN: 978-0-9964457-3-3

Library of Congress Number: 2017946495

Cover Design & Formatted

Fuzion Print - Fuzionprint.com

First printing: 2017

21 20 19 18 17   5 4 3 2 1

Table of Contents

Acknowledgments

I would like to express my sincere gratitude to the many people who supported me throughout the development of this book. To the hundreds of women who have trusted me to guide them on their health journey, it means the world to me. I am able to live my passion every day because of you. This book is dedicated to finally giving women the answers they have been searching for.

I would also like to thank Robin who helped get my ideas on paper, my editor Connie, and Ann who helped design and format this book.

Dedication

This book is dedicated to all of the women who deserve to understand their bodies and finally have answers to their years of weight loss frustrations.

About the Author

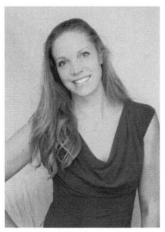

Dr. Beth Westie was born and raised on a small goat farm in Eagan, Minnesota. After collecting two state volleyball titles as an Eagan Wildcat, her sights turned to higher education in the form of becoming a NMU Wildcat. Being the recipient of a full athletic and academic scholarship to Northern Michigan University, Dr. Westie was able to combine her love of sports with her passion for women's health.

Upon graduating NMU with a bachelor's in biology and physiology, Dr. Beth Westie enrolled in the chiropractic program at Minnesota's Northwestern Health Sciences University. From there she went on to open and run a chiropractic office where she treated many women with hormone dysfunction and was able to help alleviate and resolve conditions ranging from infertility, weight gain, and inability to lose weight and keep it off, menstrual cycle issues, menopause, and more. It was then that her passion for women's health and wellness came alive, and she could transform the lives of women around the world. After selling her highly successful chiropractic practice, Dr. Westie moved full time into speaking and coaching.

In the last couple years, Dr. Westie has spent her time traveling the country, educating women and working to revolutionize the future of women's health. She has appeared on local news stations in Minnesota, Colorado, North Dakota, Virginia, Illinois, and Vermont. Dr. Westie has dedicated her life to changing the way women look at their health, and ways to effectively and safely lose weight—doing so through her customized speaking, online programs, and private coaching.

She lives in Minnesota with her husband, son, and two daughters.

To Get the Most Out of the Information in This Book

The Female Fat Solution Book was written to give you all of the basic information you need to help you understand why eating and exercising for your cycle is beneficial. I've given you all of the tools to put together a program that will help you regulate your cycle, lose weight, and improve your health. If you are like me, and want a made-for-you program specific to your body, you will want to get on the waitlist for the next 12-Week Program. In these programs, you will receive more specific guidance on how this works for you, based on your health history, hormone history, goals, dietary restrictions and more. Getting on the waitlist will give you a sneak peek at what working together looks like, and how to get started improving your health, now!

Get on the waitlist here: www.drbethwestie.com/waitlist

Part 1:

Introduction to the
Big Fat Problem

Nearly all women have been there, and if you're reading this, you probably have been, too—yo-yo dieting, nervously watching the numbers on the scale go up and down from week to week, working your butt off for months to lose weight, only to gain back the few pounds you lost.

Women have spent their time, money, and energy sweating it out, taking pills, drinking powders, fighting cravings, going hungry, and feeling the failure of trying to adapt their bodies to weight-loss plans that are not designed for women in the first place.

The big fat lie is the promise that by following a diet and exercise plan designed for men, you should get the same great results.

It's a lie. It's not true. It's never been true, and the repeated failures that women experience following this advice have only served to exacerbate the issue, eventually resulting in more serious health problems than having a little extra fat, such as diabetes, high blood pressure, heart disease, strokes, and more.

Here's the truth. It's not your fault.

These plans don't work on women's bodies because they were designed to work for men. A woman's body is not simply a smaller version of a man's. It's functionally and hormonally different. We know that, yet we continue to believe the lie, and we keep trying to force these male strategies to work with our own female bodies. Square peg, round hole, if you catch my drift.

In this book, you will learn why it is not your fault, and how you can change your approach so that it suits your own female body. Armed with knowledge on how to work *with your cycle*, and how to maximize its extremes, you can leave past "failures" behind. Delving into my program will give you a reason to feel optimistic, and be eager for a new start.

People are creatures of habit. To make a change in your body requires changing your habits. When you started a new diet or workout program in the past, you expected that you would start to develop new habits, and then two to three weeks in, or maybe even two to three months in, life happened and pulled you off track. If you weren't seeing the results you hoped for as quickly as you wanted, you may have found it even harder to stick to your new routine. If you had to count every calorie or measure every gram, you may have found staying on the program too much of a headache to stick with, so you stopped. If this happens often enough, you might even train yourself into the habit of stopping.

With my approach, which is easy enough to follow, you have no track record of failure. You can adapt it to your life no matter what's going on. Enter this process with an open mind, commitment, and some patience.

My hope is that you will read this book and become more aware of what is happening with your body, and why. You will

As soon as you "go on a diet," your body and mind are already predisposed to go off of it—unless you do something totally different.

finally have the tools you need to use your hormones to your advantage.

There is more than one path to success on my plan, and no way in order to "screw it up." You can adapt it to your life, and once and for all live a lifestyle that feels right for your body. I get asked a lot whether something is "healthy" or not. It's important to understand how much of a gray area this can be. While something might benefit one person, it might be detrimental to another, simply based on their individual body. I urge you not to look at something as healthy or unhealthy, but rather if it's going *to be beneficial for you specifically.*

Chapter 1:
The 140-Pound Man

Mary was a busy mom of three who religiously weighed herself. She was active, eating what she felt like was a clean diet, and had tried almost every known diet, but could never lose the weight she wanted. At the beginning of the program working with Dr. Beth, I took an initial weight, but then put my scale in the closet as she requested. Every week I took measurements, as well as photos to track my progress.

Not only did I almost immediately notice an increase in energy, and a much deeper sleep, I happily noted having a lot more patience with my kids. Almost every week I would message Dr. Beth saying how badly I wanted to get on the scale because I could tell things were changing, clothes were fitting differently, and I looked different.

Sure enough, at the end of week four, I couldn't believe I had gained two pounds, but I wasn't disappointed. I could not believe how good I felt, how much harder I could push myself during workouts, and best of all, I needed to buy new, smaller clothes.

-Mary, 42 years old, married, works as a
Marketing Coordinator for a corporate company.

You have tried it all. You have exercised religiously, cut carbs, and drank thick protein shakes. You have experimented with new cardio routines, strength exercises, cut out gluten and dairy, and weighed the pros and cons of veganism.

And, what do you know? After three months of this grueling effort, your favorite jeans almost zip up—but not quite. You are putting forth a consistent effort, and getting lousy results. You start to wonder if there's something wrong with you.

Then, your husband decides to jump on the bandwagon and start a diet and exercise program, maybe try a few nights a week at the gym, and skip a dessert here or a beer there. And, hey, great news! Two weeks in, he barrels into the kitchen to tell you *he's lost eight pounds*.

Sound familiar? Have you noticed, as I have, that men seem to lose weight and improve their fitness levels so much faster than women, even if the man and woman follow similar exercise and nutrition regimens. Have you ever wondered why?

Brace yourself, because when you find out, you may find it shocking.

Here's the deal. The studies and clinical trials all this mainstream advice is based upon were all done on men—and adjusted to fit women by calculating recommended dosages for a 140-pound adult male. So, almost everything you've read about calorie intake, exercise regimens, nutrient dosages, and supplements for women all are perfectly tuned to work for a 140-pound man.

How Could This Happen?

You might rightly ask how this could happen in the United States in the most scientifically advanced era in history. Until the 1990s, *women were banned* from participating in clinical trials in the U.S. [i]. According to a 2006 study in the *Journal of Women's Health*, women made up less than one-quarter of all patients enrolled in 46 examined clinical trials completed in 2004.[ii]

"Until the 1990s, women were banned from participating in clinical trials in the U.S." – Scientific American

Even more incredible, pharmaceutical companies conduct research on men to determine

Since the vast majority of research has been conducted on men, all the current mainstream recommendations that experts make regarding dietary and exercise guidelines for women are based on old data from tests done on grown men. Nowhere do they take into account women's body chemistry or the shifts and changes women experience each month.

effects of and dosages for female hormone replacement drugs. Why? It is cheaper and faster. The chemistry in a woman's body shifts so often during her lifetime that researchers would need to administer tests over a longer period of time to get accurate data. For example, a drug that causes no side effects during the first two weeks of the menstrual cycle might cause severe effects during the second two weeks.

To the pharmaceutical companies, the 140-pound male is equivalent to a 140-pound woman. Researchers take a 140-pound man and perform research on him. They do not look at how female hormones function in the female body or their cyclical fluctuations.[iii]

Additionally, scientists and clinicians tend to overlook the option of testing on female animals. According to a study in *Neuroscience and Bio-behavioral Reviews*, out of nearly 2,000 animal studies published in 2009, scientists showed a bias toward using male animals in eight of 10 disciplines.[iv]

For example, scientists dis-covered women experience greater pain relief from opioid painkillers than men do, perhaps because estrogen, which fluctuates during menstrual cycles, modulates the pain response.[v]

We know that female bodies react differently to stress. Dr. Zainab Samad, assistant professor of medicine at Duke University Medical Center in Durham, North Carolina, along with her research team, found that the effects of mental stress on the heart varied significantly

However, the little research that has been done indicates that female bodies respond differently than males'.

between men and women, according to the *Journal of the American College of Cardiology.* "This study revealed that mental stress affects the cardiovascular health of men and women differently," Dr. Samad said.[vi]

Gender Differences in Males and Females

Bottom line: female bodies react differently than male bodies because their chemistry is different, so we need to stop pretending they are the same when we prescribe diet and exercise plans.

Even from the embryologic stages of development, female bodies are put together differently than are males. While we are all aware of the obvious differences between men and women, the distinctions are more encompassing than may be outwardly apparent.

For instance:

- Men and women differ in every cell of their bodies because they carry a different chromosomal pattern.[vii]

- Women's bodies perform three very important physiological functions totally absent in men: menstruation, pregnancy, and lactation.[viii]

- Women have a larger stomach, kidneys, liver, and appendix, and smaller lungs than men.[ix]
- Gender differences become more obvious during adolescence. In females, we see increased estrogen levels and increased mass and strength of bone relative to that of muscle. In men, increases in testosterone fuel large increases in muscle mass. The result is muscle forces that coincide with a large growth in bone dimensions and strength.[x]

With all these differences, why should women follow diets, exercise routines, and lifestyle recommendations designed for men? None of it is designed for an adult female body—and it is difficult to find many resources that account for the ways a woman's body chemistry radically changes throughout her menstrual cycle, and how that affects her diet and exercise needs and outcomes.

And if we choose to follow such a plan, why would we feel like failures when men get better results? Our chemistry, our brains, our metabolism, and the way our bodies store fat, all differ from males. It makes more sense for women to follow guidelines designed especially for women.

> **No wonder women consistently get poor results with diet and exercise programs. Women have been trying to stay fit and trim by following health and fitness programs that were designed for men.**

Armed with some new insights from reading this book, you'll get the information you need to reach your goals, and begin to *work with your body's chemistry* to propel you forward into getting the results that have eluded you. You will learn to stop ignoring your menstrual cycle or viewing it as a "curse" that is holding you back, and discover how to work with your cycle to optimize your energy levels, mood, and fat loss.

Women Lose Weight Differently Than Men

One of the key things I try to stress to women is to understand that we lose weight differently than men. You may be thinking, yea, no kidding. He's in there eating pizza and drinking beer, and he's still down 10 lbs. while here I am eating my kale salad and have not lost a pound.

Here's why. When women are put into a caloric deficit, their bodies actually slow their metabolism and store every calorie as sugar in fat cells, and use muscle tissue for energy.

Have you heard of the term "skinny fat?" This is exactly what that means, and is pretty much the opposite of the overall goal.

Whereas for men, when they are put into a caloric deficit, due to testosterone they will burn fat first as energy, resulting in a shift on the scale almost immediately. Testosterone is naturally burning fat.

This is why I have a hard time with a lot of the diets targeting women. Most of the quick-fix diets are aimed at decreasing inflammation and water weight, which initially will show as the scale moving downwards. The problem with this is, as stated above, women's bodies then turn to using the muscle tissue as energy, increasing body fat percentage and overall causing women to gain weight. Women who follow this type of program are going to throw their hormones out of balance, which results in long-term repercussions for their endocrine system.

You are probably wondering then, what's the right way? So many fad diets proclaim that they help you lose weight quickly. And they might, initially. If you are looking for a long-term solution, you need to take a different approach. The woman's main focus needs to be on getting a complete nutrient meal every two to three hours. Next is increasing protein amounts, which is covered more in the next couple chapters.

What do realistic results look like for women? First, throw away your scale. I know, you've been taught to get on that thing every single morning, and you are judging your success from the day before based around that number. It's crap. It's the *worst indicator* for women in terms of success around a lifestyle change.

When women start to increase protein amounts and burn fat, the number on the scale might jump around. However, by increasing lean muscle mass, you are burning more fat and lowering your body fat percentage. Ever heard the phrase "muscle weighs more than fat?" This is where that comes in. I encourage women I work with to note things like *energy increasing, deeper sleep, less mental fog, and an ability to handle stressful situations better* as their first indicators of success. Then you can turn to using inches to determine your overall body composition changing. This is key in order for women to be set up for successful.

Side Note: When taking measurements, it's important to take measurements in a couple of different places, and here is why. Inability to lose weight in your hips and thighs can indicate a hormone imbalance, specifically for estrogen. If your trouble spot happens to be in your abdomen, this indicates a high level of cortisol. When starting out, and you're tracking progress, I encourage women to measure in these areas: arms, bust, true waist, hip, and thigh.

Female Fat Solutions:

Notice Changes in this Order:

1. Deeper sleep and increase in energy

2. Decrease in measurements

3. Decrease on the scale

Online Resources:

✓ Why The Scale Doesn't Determine Success: https://www.youtube.com/watch?v=IwNm_bmfDAY

✓ For additional FREE resources, including Recipes for Your Cycle Cookbook, Cycle Symptom Tracker and Food Habit Blueprint, visit my website: www.drbethwestie.com/resources.

Part 2:

Understanding Your Cycle

Chapter 2:
Meet "Aunt Flo" –
The 28-Day Cycle

Despite all of the crazy nicknames, Mother Nature has one purpose for your menstrual cycle, and it is serious business—to prepare your body for pregnancy.

Although this may seem like common knowledge, many women do not learn much about their cycle and ovulation until they decide to get pregnant. And even when a woman is hoping to conceive, she may simply purchase an ovulation predictor app and forego learning about her cycle, or what is actually happening in her body.

Your Period…Also Known as:
- Aunt Flo
- Your friend
- Riding the cotton pony
- Your time of the month
- Cousin Red
- Leak week
- Shark week
- The girl flu
- The red river
- On the rag

The idea of a 28-day cycle is presented as an average length. Yours may be the "31-day cycle," or the "27-day cycle," and even those numbers may vary from month to month. Many things can affect cycle length, including stress, sleep, nutrition, hormonal changes, being around other women who are of childbearing age, illness, and injury. The standard protocol is to call the first day of your period "day one." During this time, the amount of estrogen in your bloodstream will begin to rise as progesterone falls. Estrogen peaks at the point of ovulation, about two weeks into the 28- day cycle.

Ovulation is the part of the menstrual cycle when the ovaries release a mature egg, and it travels down the fallopian tube, where it waits, ready for fertilization. Typically occurring two weeks before the first day of your period, at ovulation, progesterone spikes. Therefore, ovulation marks the end of the estrogen cycle and the beginning of the next phase: the progesterone cycle.

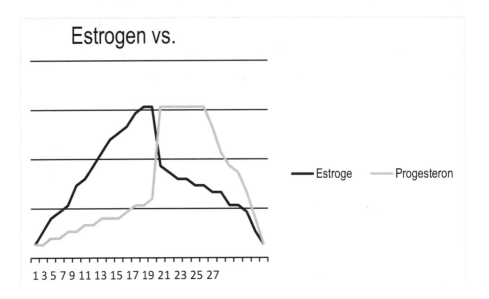

Estrogen vs.

Estroge ——— Progesteron

1 3 5 7 9 11 13 15 17 19 21 23 25 27

Tracking Ovulation

To become a slimmer, healthier you, in a way that *works with* your female body, first you've have to know how long your cycle is, and when ovulation occurs. As you will learn later, this is the key to maximizing the benefits of your nutrition and exercise efforts. It is helpful for all women to know when they ovulate because it can help you determine if your hormones are doing what they are supposed to do—flipping from estrogen dominant to progesterone dominant. If you're in your reproductive years, and they're not flipping, then something is off in your system.

Depending on which feels right for you, you can track your ovulation cycle in two different ways. Either one can work.

1) The first method is detailed and precise. Buy a thermometer and take your temperature every morning before you do anything—before you get out of bed, drink water, pee, anything—take your temperature. Write it down and then track it. Write it down on a pad of paper by your bed or put it in a spreadsheet on your computer.

First, you are looking for the lowest body temperature when you are at rest. That's what *basil body temperature* means. The hormone shifts that take place right before ovulation will cause your body temperature to decrease slightly. Then, right after ovulation, you will see a temperature spike of one-half to one degree Fahrenheit. Then your temperature will drop again. Realize, when I say "drop" it may be by only one-half of one degree. After a few weeks of tracking, you will see clear patterns. Some women may want to track their basal body temperatures for up to three months or longer, while others may want to have nothing to do with measuring and logging every morning. If that's you, I have good news.

2) The second method is a better option for those who are dismayed by the idea of charting each day. I have made this quite easy for you.

Below is a list of symptoms for the estrogen and progesterone phases of your menstrual cycle.

- **Estrogen: Day 1** – You get your period. You'll have a change in bowel movement.

- **Progesterone: Day 14** – Ovulation. Decrease in energy, cramps, slower digestive system, light cramping on one side possible, spotting, increased sense of smell and or taste, and tender breasts.
- **PMS** – Bloating, binge eating, low energy, cravings, tension, mood change, change in sleep, and a headache.

Each day, at some point, circle which of the symptoms you are experiencing. When you notice that you exhibit certain signs for three or four days in a row, you can determine whether you are in the estrogen or the progesterone phase of your cycle.

This imprecise method should not be used to help prevent or create a pregnancy, but it will give you enough information to design your nutrition and exercise plans.

For your own copy that you can print out and use over and over, go to my website, www.drbethwestie.com/resources and print out my "Cycle Symptom Tracker."

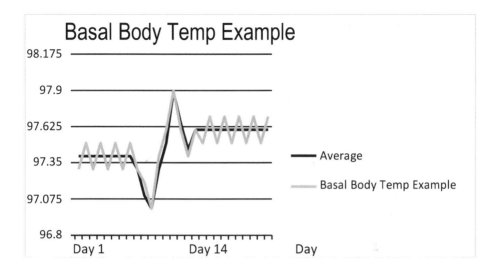

In this example, the woman's core body temperature reads 97.3, 97.5, 97.3, 97.5, 97.3, 97.5, 97.3, 97.5, then it drops to 97, spikes to 97.9 the next day and then drops to 97.4, 97.6, 97.5, 97, 97.6, 97.5, 97.6, 97.5, 97.6, 97.5, 97.6, 97.5. Ovulation occurred when the temperature dropped and then spiked.

What Does It All Mean?

Once you know when you ovulate, you can easily tell which part of the cycle you're in—whether your ovaries are pumping out estrogen to prepare for ovulation, or putting forth progesterone to prepare for pregnancy.

Now, you may wonder, "Why should I care? I mean, what does all this matter if I'm not thinking about getting pregnant?"

Here's the thing. Estrogen and progesterone affect a lot more than your uterus and ovaries. These powerful hormones also affect all the other systems in your body. And, as a result, they change how your body responds to the exercise you do, the foods you eat, and a number of other factors too numerous to name here. For this book, we will focus on the impact that estrogen and progesterone have on your metabolism, nutritional needs, and responses to exercise—*and how you can use the natural ebb and flow of these hormones to maximize your results.*

Chapter 3:
Playing with the Extremes –
Hot and Cold

For decades, health and fitness gurus have encouraged us to keep everything in balance. They say that ideal harmony is reached when two opposing sides rest on a fulcrum at an even center point, like a balance scale with each side at the same level. They say that if you follow the "middle path" and find the center between the extremes, you will attain the nirvana of balanced living.

This is a great idea—for men.

For women, this form of body balance and stability is a recipe for fat-loss failure, even if it includes exercise and "eating right"—and she needs to lean in to the extremes that each cycle presents. The female body functions best when we *increase* these natural fluctuations, and at the right times, tip the scales as far as we can in either direction.

> To devise the optimal plan for fitness and fat loss, women must view their menstrual cycle not as one singular event, but as two separate two-week phases— the "cold" estrogen cycle and the "hot" progesterone cycle.

When you're in the chilly estrogen cycle, don't try to get warm, go even *colder*. When you're in the heat of progesterone's fire, it's time to *turn it up*. The swings in your body's core temperature are designed to help your whole body function better. When you temper the extremes and move toward center stasis, you are actually hindering your female body's optimal function.

Adapt this concept to your diet and exercise plans. Forget about eating the same foods all month. Eat foods that are going to best complement your hormone levels week to week. Adapt fitness intensity to the phase you are in. Start tweaking just a few of these things from week to week and start to take note of your body's response.

A woman's body chemistry goes through radical changes throughout her menstrual cycle. You can let your menstrual cycle keep you down, or you can take advantage of the way your body's hormones naturally ebb and flow. It can limit you, or it can help. It all depends on how you look at it.

> When you learn to coordinate your diet and exercise habits with your cycle, you can optimize the weight loss and fitness benefits of exercising and eating right. You can feel better throughout the entire month, even during "that time."

Later I'm going to explain exactly how, like hundreds of women already have, you can use your cycle to help optimize not only fat loss, but also your performance and results in every area of your life. You will learn how to make the most of the gift that nature has given you. You will come to see that your menstrual cycle truly is your "friend."

Chapter 4:
Exercise with Your Cycle

Syncing your exercise and activity allows you to take advantage of the hormone cycle your body goes through each month.

- During the first week of your cycle, and this is the start of the period, women are often told to "suck it up" when they are feeling subpar or having symptoms. You are told, "Get to the gym" and start exercising to release endorphins to improve how you are feeling—but are told nothing about shifting the activity to match what is occurring in the body at that time. During the first week, it can be helpful to do lighter workouts than you would normally do until you feel you can push your body. Exercise like walking, yoga, or swimming can be beneficial at this time.

- During the second week of the cycle is often when women have the most energy all month, so push your routine during this time. High Intensity Interval Training (HIIT) is beneficial during this time. Estrogen relaxes smooth muscles so pushing your endurance now will feel easier to accomplish. Watching your form during this time is crucial because the increase in estrogen increases flexibility, and you have a higher risk of injury.

- During the third week of the cycle, energy starts to decline slightly, and it can feel like more of a struggle to get through a workout. Flexibility declines some, but you can still push more in a workout.

- During the fourth week of the cycle, some symptoms may start to pop up, so lighten your workouts somewhat, and it is very beneficial to complete your workouts in the morning due to energy levels declining a lot throughout the day.

Chapter 5:
The Estrogen Phase

My biggest vice before starting this was sugar, especially a week before my cycle would start. Amazing how eating the right foods eliminated those cravings. Excited to continue this journey and to see how my body starts changing on the outside, too.

— Taylor, 31 years old, single, works as an
Administrative Assistant.

We will start with *estrogen*, which dominates the first two weeks of an average menstrual cycle. Estrogen is a generic term for three female sex hormones: estrone, estradiol, and estriol. The ovaries are the primary producers of estrogen, however it is also produced by fat cells and the adrenal gland. Estrogen levels build during the first half of the menstrual cycle until ovulation, and then estrogen drops.

Volumes of books are devoted to the various roles estrogen plays in women's bodies, but you should know that estrogen lowers core body temperature, burns carbs, increases metabolism, and increases flexibility.

One could say that estrogen equals energy. The two weeks of the estrogen part of your menstrual cycle tend to be peak-energy times. You can use this energetic part of your cycle to plan high-activity days, and to tackle challenges that require more energy.

> **During the estrogen phase,
> it's important to keep everything cool.**

- During the first two weeks of your cycle, while estrogen and energy are on the rise, your body temperature drops. To squeeze more out estrogen in this energetic part of your cycle, and to get lean, bring your body temperature down as low as possible. Estrogen helps the body burn more carbohydrate as well. Eating foods that are cooling, as well as consuming cool beverages, will help you take advantage of your body's carb-burning properties during this time.

- During this phase, you will notice an increase in mental focus, which makes it a great time to begin a new habit. You are much more likely to stick with something that you start during the first two weeks of your cycle.

Nutrition

In the estrogen phase, in addition to consuming cooling foods, I recommend carb cycling, which will include some low-to-no carb days. Carbohydrate cycling is basically an eating plan where you choose to vary your level of carb intake from day to day. For example, with carb cycling you might consume 200 grams of carbs one day, 150 grams the next, then 50 grams the next, before starting over again. When I talk about carbohydrates, I am referring to all carbohydrate intake for the day, including starches such as potatoes, rice, oatmeal and bread. Some fruits and vegetables are carbohydrates as well, and I also recommend counting them in total intake.

Carb cycling works by tricking your body into burning fat. The body is designed to be very adaptive. It wants to recognize any patterns within a few days, and alter the regulating systems to those patterns. Your body gets accustomed to certain foods and activities, and will store more calories from food and burn fewer calories from the workouts. For instance, your body treats all sugars equally, whether they are from a candy bar, pizza dough, or an orange. When you eat about the same number of carbs per day, your body grows accustomed to them, so it stores the "energy," otherwise known as calories. This is why experts recommend varying both your food and exercise. You have to constantly and consistently change up your workout and nutrition patterning so your body doesn't adapt. By eating increased carbs for a couple of days, your body thinks that's the new "norm," and will rev up the carbohydrate-burning mode, but a couple of days later you drop the carb intake and the body is burning carbs at an all-time high. By the time the body tries to adapt and slow the carb burning, you are back to eating a higher amount again, and your body will continue to burn carbs at a high level.

Stay one step ahead of your body and in control of how its running, instead of being one step behind — and reacting.

Carb Cycling Examples:	
Example 1:	**Example 2:**
Day 1: 200g	Day 1: 200g
Day 2: 150g	Day 2: 50g
Day 3: 100g	Day 3: 125g
Day 4: 50g	Day 4: 200g
Day 5: 125g	Day 5: 50g
Day 6: 200g	Day 6: 125g
Day 7: 150g	Day 7: 200g
* Repeat	* Repeat

The only time a woman might feel uncomfortably cold during the estrogen cycle is when she is carb cycling and has a low-to-no carb day. She will feel colder because she simply does not have as many sugars in her body to burn as quickly because she has not been eating as many carbs.

Carbohydrate Amounts in Common Foods:

- Bagel (one whole) = 45g
- Bread (one slice) = 15g
- 1 cup rice = 45g
- 1 cut pasta = 40g
- ½ cup quinoa = 20g
- Popcorn (3 cup air popped) = 20g
- Glass of wine = 5g
- Apple = 22g
- Orange = 21g
- Banana = 30g
- Raw carrot = 8g
- Sweet potato = 25g
- 1 cut oatmeal = 27g

One of my favorite client stories based around carb cycling is about Julie. She came to me wanting to lose over 100 pounds, but wanted to start off with something she could realistically stick to. So of course I met her where she was at, and decided to start with carb cycling. We adapted the plan to fit her lifestyle, and set short-term, attainable goals. She used an app to log her carb amounts until she got a better handle on gauging it herself.

After 90 days Julie had lost 27 pounds, and after 11 months she was nearing her overall goal of 100 pounds.

Foods to Focus on During the Cooling Phase:

- Chicken, turkey, and fish

- Raw fruits and vegetables

- Beverages that are room temp or below

- The less caffeine and sugar the better

- Seasonings and spices: cumin, basil, parsley, sage, rosemary, thyme, coriander, fennel, mint, saffron, dill

- Limit dairy

Other Ways to Enhance the Cooling Properties of Estrogen

Using peppermint oil or a cream with peppermint oil can help cool down the body. Taking a cooler shower, or being in a cooler environment can also help you achieve the benefits of the estrogen phase.

Exercise During the Estrogen Phase

During the first two weeks of your cycle, it's important to focus on ramping up intensity, flexibility, and endurance. Estrogen is on the rise, which brings you more energy and increases your metabolism. It is easier for your body to recover, allowing you to push yourself harder. If you want to increase weight or repetitions, have at it. This is the perfect time for that.

Heart-Rate focus: Anaerobic Zone (80-90% of Heart-rate max)

Workouts I would recommend: Weight lifting, HIIT, cardio, yoga, Pilates

Chapter 6:
The Progesterone Phase

During the second half of your menstrual cycle, after you ovulate, estrogen dips as *progesterone* levels spike. Progesterone is produced in the ovaries and adrenal glands. Its role is to stimulate the uterus to prepare for pregnancy. During the progesterone phase, your core body temperature goes up, and the "internal switch" flips. When your core body temperature increases, it's important to consume warming foods and beverages during this time to increase those fat-burning properties.

Increased progesterone levels also turn on the fat-burning mode.

Carbs and Progesterone

During the second half of your cycle, you should consume carbs at a consistent amount. How many carbs you will consume daily is going to depend on your height, weight, and fitness level. For a woman of average height and weight who is working out 3–4 times per week, a good number to aim for is 125g of carbs per day.

Fasting/Cleanse Day

During the progesterone phase, I recommend a day of fasting or cleansing, once during each of those two weeks.

Historically, many different cultures have practiced fasting. It is not a new concept, but a lot of people don't understand the benefits it has for the body. Benefits include a boosted immune system, a boosted digestive system function, increased metabolism, and it boosts human growth hormone in women by 1300%, and more.

The fasting day will consist of a limited calorie intake. You would consume between 400–500 calories throughout the day. The snacks need to consist of quality food with protein, carbs, and fat. Almonds are a great example of a snack for a fasting day. Aim for having 5 snacks consisting of 80–100 calories per snack.

During the first eight hours of your fast, your body is going to burn through your stored glycogen—using up all of your stored carbohydrate as energy. Once you pass the eight-hour mark, you may begin to feel hungry because by mid-afternoon you have depleted the sugars in your body. It is at this point that your body starts burning visceral fat. You are in this deep-fat burning zone for the rest of the day, or until your break your fast. Maintaining a long-term (longer than 72 hours/3 days) low-caloric diet is not advised. At this point, your body will begin attacking muscle tissue and proteins in the body to use as energy, breaking down muscle fibers and connective tissue. Maintaining a fast longer than 72 hours will slow down your metabolism.

I had been working with Jessie for two months. She had tried a couple different cleanses in the past, but was hesitant to try one with me. I assured her it wasn't the same as what she had tried in the past, and we would be incorporating small snacks throughout the day. She trusted me and tried it for 24 hours. I set her up on a proper protocol, and was excited to see her results the next day.

Here is what she had to say: "Dr. Beth, I cannot believe how much energy I have. It's like I'm in hyper drive. My focus is incredible, I woke up before my alarm today, and I was shocked at how easy yesterday was. I never really felt hungry, I stuck to the plan, stayed busy and drank a lot of water. Today I'm down 3 pounds, and 2 inches off my waist"

Anytime you are in contact with toxins, whether it be chemical, environmental, something you breathe, or something you eat, the toxins and excess hormone get stored in the visceral fat cells. Another important benefit of fasting is that it helps release toxins and built-up hormone that is stored, allowing your liver to process it and release it from the body.

So let's talk a little bit about fat cells. A lot of misconceptions exist around fat cells, so let's set a few things straight. First off, you have the same amount of fat cells now as you did when you were born. You might be thinking, okay, but then how does someone "lose weight." Think of your fat cells like a flat pancake, or at least that's what they're supposed to look like. When estrogen, progesterone, cortisol, and adrenaline are stored inside the fat cells, they blow up like a balloon. This is what causes people to look like they have gained weight.

> **Going through a fat-cell cleanse to help release that excess hormone from the fat cell is vital to losing weight and visceral fat.**

The Heat Is on

During the progesterone phase you want to be sure to complement the warming properties with more warming-focus foods.

Foods to Focus on Eating During the Warming Phase:

- Spicy food will heat up your system.

- Peppers bring more physical heat into the body, warming up your digestive system, which is closely connected with your endocrine system.

- Red meats, such as beef and bacon, are warming for the body.

- Nightshade vegetables (vegetables that grow at night), such as tomatoes, eggplant, paprika, pimentos, hot peppers and sweet peppers all bring the heat.

- Hot drinks such as hot water with lemon, tea or coffee warm you up. Caffeine brings extra heat to the body, too, so if you want a second cup of coffee during this time, go ahead and have it.

- Seasonings and spices: cinnamon, cloves, nutmeg, cayenne, paprika, garlic, onion, red pepper, ginger, turmeric

- Avoid peanuts during Week 4. Your gall bladder function is decreased during this week, and peanuts will aggravate it further.

Other Ways to Bring the Heat

Adding heat during your progesterone phase is not limited to what you put inside your body. Warm up your body with hot baths and showers, or by bundling up and relaxing next to a warm fire.

Exercise During the Progesterone Phase

During the last two weeks of your cycle, it's important to focus on getting into the fat-burning zone. Focusing more on cardio in this phase will help you utilize the fat-burning properties of progesterone. It's the perfect time to increase sets if you are lifting weights.

Heart-rate focus: Aerobic zone (70-80% of HR Max).

Workouts I would recommend: Cardio, HIIT, weight lifting

Keep the Main Thing the Main Thing

If you LOVE to do something when it comes to exercising, do that! You are much more likely to stick to something you love. When we talk about shifting your exercise to match your cycle, focus more on intensity. I'm not going to tell you one week to go to Yoga, and then take up bodybuilding the next, and by the end of the month make sure you are signed up to run a marathon. NO! Whatever you are into, keep that the main thing. Focus more on the intensity of the activity you are doing. Adjust your effort to match the phase you are in, and you will be well on your way to using your cycle to your advantage.

Chapter 7:
Planning Nutrition Cycles

Week 1 **&** **Week 2**	• Everything should be cooling and calm • <u>Focus Foods:</u> RAW Vegetables, Chicken, Fish, Fruits, lukewarm and cold drinks, smaller amounts of coffee and tea • --Limit Dairy • --Carb Cycling can be added. • Example 1: M: 200g T: 150g W: 100g Th: 50g Fri: 125g S: 150g Sun: 200g
Week 3 **&** **Week 4**	• Focus on warming and extra Fat in the morning • <u>Focus Foods:</u> All foods should be COOKED, Red meat, bacon, night shade—tomatoes, peppers, HOT coffee and tea. • DECREASE peanut intake • --Add Dairy Back in • --Add one cleanse day this week

Female Fat Solutions:

1. During the estrogen phase, keep every cool and add in carb cycling.
2. During the progesterone phase, keep everything warm, and add in fasting.
3. Find an activity you love doing, and focus on altering your heart rate for each phase.

Videos:

- ✓ How to Use Estrogen to Lose Weight!
  https://www.youtube.com/watch?v=lDgB6qLn65o

- ✓ How to Use Progesterone to Lose Weight:
  https://www.youtube.com/watch?v=GJwu8pD9frE

- ✓ Want to Eat More Carbs?
  https://www.youtube.com/watch?v=f16TohZuL4A

- ✓ Fat Cell Secrets! What they are and how to shrink them:
  https://www.youtube.com/watch?v=UaywEsthLjE

Part 3:

Nutrition Basics for Women

Before you dive into any kind of plan, its important to have a good idea of basic nutrition. You need to know the basics of what a *macro* versus *micronutrient* is. If you follow me on social media, I tell my followers to make sure they are having complete nutrient snacks and meals. That means having a protein, fat, and carb incorporated in every meal or mini meal you eat. In order to start building complete nutrient meals it's important to understand each component.

Chapter 8:

Know What to Eat—

and Not to Eat, and When

I was desperate for something to help me get through my workday without needing an energy drink or cup of coffee midafternoon. Some days I felt like the energy drink or coffee was making me even more tired. Per Dr. Beth's advice, I added 2 tablespoons of coconut oil to my coffee in the morning, and to make some fat bombs to eat around lunchtime. The FIRST day I noticed a difference. After a week I had overcome that midafternoon crash, and now have more energy than I had felt in a long time.

> – Jennifer, 33 year old, married, mom of
> 1 works as an Account Manager.

> **Complete nutrient snacks and meals means having a protein, fat, and carb incorporated in every meal or mini meal you eat.**

The body burns the nutrient in your food in a specific order After eating, your body use the carbohydrate as energy within the first hour. During the next two to three hours, it turns over to using protein, and lastly at the four-hour mark, it begins to use fat as energy.

Yes, it can be confusing when I use the term fat, and you may be thinking fat on your body, but for this I am talking about the nutrient fat. When we talk about getting to the point where your body uses fat for fuel, it's essentially depleted, thus slowing down your metabolism. It doesn't have any additional fuel source stored up, and is waiting for the next nutrient source.

My client, Sarah, is a busy teacher in a kindergarten classroom. She was eating breakfast around 6:30 a.m., and was not able to get in any nutrient until her lunch around 12:30. Overall she felt like she was eating a clean diet, and exercising, but was not getting the results she was seeking, and noticed her energy crashing around 2 p.m. By simply adding in a protein bar, cut up into 8 small pieces that she could easily grab frequently throughout the day, she was well on her way to reaching her goals. By keeping her metabolism going throughout the day, it helped her get back on track.

After only four weeks of doing this Sarah noticed a massive increase in her energy in the afternoon, she had lost 6 inches, and was down 4 pounds.

It's important to eat more frequently as a tactic to increase the rate at which your metabolism burns. Never go longer than three hours between meals or mini meals. If you have reached the four-hour mark, and you haven't eaten any nutrient, you are essentially killing your metabolism. Think of it like refueling a car. The four-hour mark represents being out of gas and stranded. If you don't want to be stuck on the side of the road, make sure you are eating a complete nutrient every two to three hours.

Protein: When Life Gives You Lemons, Ask for Something Higher in Protein

Protein is an essential building block for muscles and cells. Every cell in your body requires protein to function. It is also essential for muscle function and to maintain lean body mass. For women it's tougher to build lean muscle than it is for men, which is where protein comes in to play. And let me be clear that I'm not talking about "bulking up," which is a huge misconception when increasing protein amounts in your diet. It's vital for women to be getting an appropriate amount of protein and in the right form in order to increase lean muscle mass, and in turn, burn fat.

Women have a different muscle composition than men, so it is especially important to get more protein. Unfortunately, women do not naturally build lean muscle as quickly as men. Muscle tissue in women has a completely different composition. Even when you increase protein in women, although the body is less likely to use muscle tissue as fuel, they will still build lean muscle at a slower rate.

> **Women do not get enough protein in their diet in general, which leads to their body using muscle tissue as fuel.**

There are numerous other benefits of increasing protein amounts in your diet. Some include increased energy, better sleep, less mental fog, weight loss, less joint pain, stronger hair and nails, firmer skin, and a better response to stress.

Forms of Healthy Proteins:

- Grass-fed beef

- Organic poultry

- Wild-caught fish

- Undenatured whey protein

- Nuts

- Seeds

- Cottage cheese

- Greek yogurt

- Plant-based protein free of soy

- Organic cage-free eggs

- Beans (garbanzo, kidney, black, legumes)

Carbohydrates: Meet Your New BFF – Carbs

> **These systems run off of carbohydrate. When you deplete these systems of the fuel they need to properly function, it throws off their ability to release and regulate hormone.**

Carbs get a very bad rap, and it's unfortunate. Lots of low- or no-carb diets will provide an initial result, but are very damaging long term for women. Here is why. Your brain and nervous system control the release of hormone in the body and help regulate hormones. This is why it is vital for women to make sure they are incorporating a healthy amount of carbohydrate in their daily diets.

In the estrogen chapter I will dive into carb cycling and how changing the amount of carb you are eating daily during the first two weeks of your cycle can ignite your metabolism and help your body to burn those carbs.

To be totally transparent, different types of carbs will have a different affect on the body and blood sugar. Low-glycemic carbs have a lower sugar content per serving than a high glycemic. Pineapples are high glycemic, while strawberries are low glycemic. Therefore, eating a couple slices of pineapple is going to spike and then drop your blood sugar on a much larger scale than a cup of berries would.

I do recommend a complete nutrient to help combat this blood sugar spike and drop. If you are to consume a cup of berries, pairing it with a handful of almonds, your blood sugar would go up slightly, but the protein and fat in the almonds would help it level off instead of dropping. Another benefit of making sure all of your meals contain some carb is added energy. Having more energy can help push yourself harder during your workouts, in turn helping you reach your goals faster.

Forms of Healthy Carbohydrate

- Lentils

- Quinoa

- Brown rice

- Fruit

- Sweet potatoes

- Potatoes

- Gluten-free pasta

- Gluten-free bagel/bread

- Steel-cut oats

Fats: Fat Does NOT Make You Fat

We've all heard the old wives' tale that eating fat will make you fat—which is so far from the truth it's almost kind of funny. Omega 3 Fats are essential for key systems in your body, including your nervous system, brain function, and cardiovascular function. At the same time, they play a vital role in leveling out your blood sugars. Without fat in your diet, your cells, your brain, and your nervous system are unable to function optimally. When cutting out fats, women may notice more brain fog, mental fatigue, and their energy crashing midafternoon. Fats play a very important role in healthy hair, skin, and nails. If you want to have strong nails and glowing skin, add some healthy fats.

Here is an example of a fat bomb. Having two to four fat bombs per day is a great alternative when you are feeling like you need a snack or a sweet treat.

Lemon Fat Bomb

Ingredients:
- 4 Tbsp grass-fed butter (I like Kerrygold)
- 4 Tbsp coconut oil
- 2 oz cream cheese
- 1 scoop vanilla protein powder

Directions:
1. Warm and melt butter, coconut oil, and cream cheese.
2. Mix in protein, add a splash of water if needed.
3. Mix in lemon flavor and place in 2 Tbsp in ice cube tray or in cupcake wrappers.
4. Freeze for 4 hours. Enjoy!

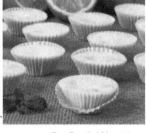

Dr. Beth Westie

You can find more fat bomb recipes, including my personal favorite, chocolate peanut butter, in my cookbook! Go to www.drbethwestie.com/resources to grab your copy!

People are still buying into the idea of eating low fat, or drinking diet soda as being healthier for you than full-fat options. Marketing can cause a lot of confusion when it comes to what is and what is not actually healthy for the body. Companies market this way because the calorie count on the label is going to be lower than the full-fat version. However, when you look at the density in a nutrient versus calorie amount, you are actually looking at the fuel your body is going to gain from a specific food source. We are talking about *quality over quantity* here.

Fats help you absorb fat-soluble vitamins like vitamin A, E, D, and K. This is why people on a low fat diet find themselves being deficient in these main categories, which can result in disease, decreased healing time, and decreased immune function.

Forms of Healthy Fats

- Coconut oil
- Olive oil
- Avocado
- Avocado oil
- Sunflower oil
- Safflower oil
- Walnuts
- Almond
- Pecans
- Butter from grass-red cows
- Omega 3s

Micronutrients = Vitamins and Minerals

Micronutrients are required for normal growth and development of living organisms. Vitamins and minerals are essential to have in your daily diet. The food that is produced today has less nutrient and minerals available than there was fifty years ago, making it vital to supplement with additional vitamins and minerals to be sufficient. Most women are lacking in vital nutrients and minerals because of this depletion in the soil.

Minerals are necessary for proper building of bone, teeth, blood, skin, hair, nails, and nerve function. Additionally, they are vital for the metabolic process that converts food to energy. Therefore, an increase in minerals equals an increase in energy. If you are deficient in vitamins and minerals, *you increase your chance for disease.*

Chapter 9
Nutrition Fundamentals—
What's "Fun" About
Fundamentals

Avoid Dairy, Gluten, and Other Inflammatory Foods

I ate a very clean diet, and exercised 5 days per week. I contacted Dr. Beth, wanting to get rid of my belly bloat. Feeling like I was doing all the right things, I couldn't understand why it never seemed to go away, and on some days was bad enough to make me "look 4 months pregnant." Dr. Beth suggested I try cutting out dairy to see if that would have any effect. One week in…and I couldn't believe it. Belly bloat was gone. I was so amazed that one small tweak could make such a huge difference.

– Susan, 45 and active

Eliminating inflammatory foods from your diet is beneficial in numerous ways. Every disease that your body can get is linked to inflammation, so there is real value in reducing the inflammatory foods. This will significantly reduce your chances of getting seriously ill—and you will notice more energy, less puffiness, and fewer digestive issues.

Going Gluten Free

We all have that friend who decided to "go gluten free" in order to lose weight. And maybe at first that worked, but having done only a little research, she cooked everything from a box, and soon saw her results head the opposite direction.

So what is it about gluten that you should avoid, and how can it benefit some people?

Gluten is very inflammatory in the body. The way gluten is produced in the United States has made it become very inflammatory, especially in the digestive system. Therefore, when someone decides to cut gluten from her diet, she is going to reduce inflammation and allow the body to process and digest food more optimally. You are better able to absorb the nutrient you are eating, and will experience less digestive issues. Going gluten free will get you a better result—but may not be for everyone. I highly encourage you to make sure you do your research on this before you dive in.

> The goal of going gluten free would be to cut a lot of processed junk out of your diet, and embark on eating more naturally.

The Dairy Dilemma

Eliminating dairy from your diet is not as straightforward. Basically, it is a bit of trial-and-error to determine what your body will tolerate. Dairy is inflammatory, but delivers many healthy nutrients to your body. Some people, especially those who have gout or rheumatoid arthritis, may feel better if they cut out dairy completely. Others can handle yogurts and cheeses because they are more processed, and the proteins are more broken down so they are easier to digest. And not all cheeses are created equally. Maybe you think your body does not respond well to cheese, but what quality of cheese did you buy? Make sure you buy high-quality products to put into your body. For instance, high-quality mozzarella cheese has a ton of protein, and is easier to digest than the less-expensive stuff.

A lot of confusion exists around dairy versus lactose. *Lactose* is sugar found in milk. Often when people think they have an issue with dairy, it's not actually the dairy that is the problem, but the lactose. In humans, around age 5 we lose an enzyme that allows us the ability to process lactose. Therefore, having lactose after this age, people might see symptoms like bloating, gas, or other digestive issues.

Hard cheeses and yogurt, for example, do not contain lactose, but are considered dairy. You can see how this might be confusing. Someone might not have any issues with hard cheese or yogurt, but experience immense digestive issues with milk.

> A lot of times when people think they have an issue with dairy, it's not actually the dairy that is the problem, but the lactose.

When you are debating whether or not to cut dairy, first experiment with what might work best for you. Many people periodically eliminate and then re-introduce dairy, or they limit daily and weekly servings. Even cutting down on the amount of dairy you consume, as well as consuming higher-quality dairy, will provide you with a positive result.

Eat More Leafy Green Veggies Daily

Did you know it takes 50 bowls of spinach today to equal one bowl of spinach from 1950? People miss out on eating the nutrients they need, then overeat the junk they don't need, like chips and donuts. Did you ever hear someone say, "Oh, I overdid it on my greens today." Let's admit it, people don't overeat greens.

We are eating too much junk. That's one reason that I preach *organic*. With organic produce, you are going to get more of the nutrients that you need. Organic food is not genetically modified, with no pesticides or other chemicals. It is simply pure, wholesome food. And, with the stressful lifestyles we lead, the disease and environmental toxins your body has to fight, give your body more nutrients than what the government recommends. If you do, you will be much better armed to fight off the things that are not good for you.

At home, I use a blend of greens. I'll purchase a bag of mixed greens and throw them in my blender. An easy way to add greens is to juice them and add them to an ice cube tray. Then the greens are ready whenever you need them. An easy way to incorporate them is by putting the ice cubes in your shake or smoothie.

Benefits of Eating Organic:

You may have noticed I recommend things like grass-fed butter and beef, or free-range organic chicken, or cage-free eggs. Are you wondering why?

- It is more environmentally friendly to eat organic.

- In byproducts from grass-fed animals, a fatty acid, CLA, has been shown to burn more fat naturally in your body.

- In organic products, there is more nutrient component to the product.

- Organic products also have less chemicals and antibiotics.

Limit Sugar and Salt—Too much sugar and salt are bad for your body, yet sugar and salt are essential to a properly functioning body. The key is moderation. The typical person is getting enough sugar from her daily diet. If there's too much sugar in your diet, it can be very addictive. Scientists have found that sugar has a powerful effect on the reward centers of the brain, creating a similar response in those parts of the brain as addictive drugs, such as cocaine and nicotine.

Most bottled beverages often contain excess sugar to make it taste better, urging you to drink more. This being said, it's important to watch for this in anything you drink from a bottle. For example, in one serving (8 oz.) of Minute Maid Orange Juice you will consume 24g of sugar. In one serving of Lipton Iced Tea (8 oz.), you are consuming 21g of sugar.

Too much salt can have a negative impact on your blood pressure, kidneys, insulin resistance, and more. Already so much salt is added to processed food, you must be careful about adding more.

However, let's see the other side to this. While both fast food and processed food contain a lot of excess sodium, if you are cooking your meals yourself, adding a little extra salt can actually be beneficial. Salt is a necessary mineral to have in your diet at some level. Himalaya and sea salt are healthier versions because they aren't processed or acid-washed. Iodine in salts is vital for thyroid function and avoiding goiters, which is a bigger problem for those living in the Midwest due to lack of seafood.

Avoid Over-processed Foods—I know you are thinking pretty much everything in the 27 aisles of the grocery store is processed, so how are you supposed to avoid this? Let me explain. Technically peanut butter is processed, but you are better off if you buy organic peanut butter with only peanuts and salt being listed in the ingredients.

**The more natural and closer to original form,
the more nutrient your body can absorb from it.**

The more systems it has to go through to be broken down in different forms, the harder it is for your body to break it down and absorb the most nutrient from it.

Start shopping for your groceries by going around the outside aisles. Pick up your organic fruits and veggies first, and then move onto your grass-fed beef and organic poultry. Avoiding buying most of your groceries as things in a box.

Sweet Rewards

I don't use the term, "cheat meals," and here's why. Life is about balance. When we use the term "cheat" it seems like you are doing something negative. I firmly believe that if you want to have the piece of cake at your kid's birthday party, you should have it; however, don't dive into an entire pie every day. The more you restrict yourself, the harder it is to make an overall lifestyle change. If you allow yourself those small things you want every now and again, you are less likely to completely fall off the bandwagon.

Another strategy with sweet treats is to find ways to make your favorites a little bit healthier. I love using protein powder to make some of my favorite treats, like donuts, protein balls, and muffins.

You can find more of my favorite recipes in my High Protein & Fat Bomb Recipe Book. Go to www.drbethwestie.com/resources to grab your copy!

Read the Label—I'm not talking about reading the nutrient content listed on the label, but reading the ingredients in the product. It's important to know what hidden ingredients or foods that are misrepresented, in other words, be able to spot the junk. There are a lot of loopholes in food production, and if you are not aware of what to be on the lookout for, it can be sabotaging your results.

Some things to watch for: Hydrogenated oil, artificial sweeteners (aspartame), fillers (cellulose powder), colors/dyes, coatings on food, to name a few.

Stay Hydrated—You literally cannot live without water. We know this, but many of us do not get nearly the amount of water we need each day. So why is water vital to life?

You need it to detoxify your body, digest food, dissolve nutrients, and much more. How much should you be drinking each day? It's all depends on your activity level. A good benchmark is to drink a gallon on days you are active or working out, and a half gallon on other days.

Being dehydrated has a plethora of negative health implications. For instance, toxins will remain in your body longer, it will be harder to digest food, and your organs will have to work harder to function properly. If the lymphatic system doesn't have enough fluid, it's not going to pump nutrients to the body as efficiently.

When people get dehydrated, they often don't recognize it because we most often associate thirst with dehydration, when in reality we know many other symptoms.

Headaches are a very common symptom of dehydration. A lot of people will feel ill, and get flu-like symptoms. I've been dehydrated before when I was younger, and my first symptom was stomach pain. I'd do my chores in the morning, play outside, and then ride bikes with my friends. I never took a water bottle with me. Here I was, a little girl on the go all day long, and I did not hydrate/drink water at all. Periodically I'd end up with severe stomach pain—dehydration.

Watch Portion Sizes—I remember going to my grandmother's house for a meal, and she would set the whole table, a plate for the main course, a smaller plate, a glass for water and a tiny glass for juice. The plate for the main course looked like what we use for a salad plate today. The juice glasses were my favorite because they were small and cute.

Today, plates are huge and cups are enormous. Many of the messages telling you to eat more come from external cues, not your body. As a result, we have people packing their plates full or food, and filling up a hi-ball glass with juice, which contains at least five servings. People don't think about how much food they load onto a plate, and then they feel guilty if they don't eat every bite. Think of the "clean-plate award" your parents might have given out.

The size of our portions here in the U.S. is out of control both at restaurants and in our homes.

Let's use pasta as an example. You've probably been to a restaurant before and ordered a plate of spaghetti. Out comes a plate piled high with pasta, spaghetti sauce, and meatballs. However, when you check out the pasta package you might cook at home, you may be shocked to find out that a serving size is only ¾ cup. Now let's look back at the serving you received at the restaurant which might have been 4 to 5 times that, and most likely you ate all of it. You can see what I mean when I say our portion sizes are out of control.

The other part of the problem is that people eat all this food, drink all these juice and soda. Then, an hour later, guess what? Hungry again. Why is that? It's mostly due to the lack of nutrient in our food and drink. The body isn't getting the nutrient it needs—and is asking for more.

> **A lot of times when people think they have an issue with dairy, it's not actually the dairy that is the problem, but the lactose.**

People tend to panic a little when I bring up portion control, but here's the secret. When you eat a balanced diet of complete nutrients, frequently (every 2–3 hours), you won't feel deprived or hungry. For example, if I suggest making a protein pancake, they aren't even tempted to eat a giant stack of six. One or two is enough, and my clients feel satisfied.

Nutrition and Mindset
The reason for making a lifestyle change has to be bigger than a number.

When it comes to starting a new program or adopting a healthier lifestyle, it's important that at the same time, you work on your mindset around nutrition.

When you start something new, it's essential to know exactly *why you are doing it.* If you dig deep and find the true reason you want to make a change, you are much more likely to stick to a plan that will get you there. Now I know "to lose weight" might seem like the obvious answer. But I want you to dig deeper. What will that weight loss do for you? Will you have more energy to play with your kids? Maybe you want to run a 5k. Or maybe it's for a different health reason. Whatever it is, find your why and write it down, or find a picture that represents it. Keep it somewhere that you will see it every single day.

Often women have tried numerous programs in the past, and usually have a set point at which they "fail" or give up.

Whether that is 5 days or 5 weeks, it is still a set point, meaning you are highly likely to quit any new program that you start at this exact same point. However, once you are aware of this set point, you can change it by building strategies around this time in order to keep moving forward.

The answers to these questions will give you your *food habit blueprint.* What habits did you grow up around when it comes to food?

- How do you shop for food?
- How do you prepare food?

- How do you eat food?
- What amount of food do you put on your plate?
- How do you feel about food?
- When do you eat?

What do I mean by this, and why is it so important? All of us grew up with different ideas and habits formed around food—some good, some not so good.

I love to tell this story: When a woman was preparing a roast for her family, she proceeded to cut off the end. Her daughter asked why she had to cut off the end, and she said because that's how her mom did it. So the girl went to ask her grandma why she cut the end off her roast, and she told her because that's what her mom did. Then the girl went to ask her great grandma why she cut off the end off her roast. Her answer: because her oven was too small to fit the whole thing.

Now this might be funny, but it goes to show a lot about how we develop habits. We tend to adapt behaviors from our parents without ever asking why. The majority of your food-habit blueprint was probably based on the way your parents did things.

Did you know that back in the 1960s and '70s, as things like the microwave and dishwasher were being developed, food was also being changed to become more "convenient." No laws on how food was advertised were in place so a lot of misrepresentation occurred when it came to "healthy" food.

The FDA didn't regulate it, so companies were putting labels on foods and calling them healthy, when in fact they weren't. It's important to take a step back and truly understand what your blueprint is, and where you want it to be. If you aren't happy with where your relationship is with food now, *then it's time to change it.*

Female Fat Solutions:

1. Make sure every meal or mini meal is a complete nutrient.
2. Implement a lifestyle change instead of a fad diet.
3. Work on your "Mindset Around Nutrition" in order to develop your own.

Go to my website: www.drbethwestie.com and get your Food Habit Blueprint

Videos:

✓ How is Protein Absorbed in the Body?: https://www.youtube.com/watch?v=UhGeGJrpLvw
✓ Why are Carbs so Important: https://www.youtube.com/watch?v=ZyTiRLnMqQY
✓ Healthy Fats Won't Make You Fat and Here's Why!: https://www.youtube.com/watch?v=k0bazmDsxMw
✓ What is Soil Depletion & Why are Supplements Important: https://www.youtube.com/watch?v=MmyKufLDy-Y

Part 4:

Exercise Basics for Women

Chapter 10:
Getting Started — Overall
Approach to Exercise

I had been working with Dr. Beth on my nutrition for a couple of months, and I was feeling so much better that I wanted to add in a different form of exercise. I had never belonged to a gym, nor ever lifted a weight, and I really didn't want to start there. Dr. Beth suggested I join her Boot Camp class to see what I thought. I was hooked after the first day. It was an all-female gym full of supportive women. Quickly I became friends with them, and in two weeks, I was asking women from the class to join me for a 5k. It was incredible how quickly I found her groove—and something I loved. I won't be giving that up anytime soon.

– Jen, 35-year-old, married mom of 2, works
as a Speech Pathologist.

Exercise recommendations have been researched by men—and the programs were created for men. Only in recent decades have women been even allowed to participate in sports. And videos of women "exercising" from the 1950s showed them pretty much laying on weird roller machines while wearing heels and in full makeup. Women were thought to be too fragile for any hearty activity as it would somehow damage their delicate being. If only we could lie on roller machines and get fit, right?

You might have flashbacks to gym classes of the past, being forced to participate wearing hideous clothing and being embarrassed in front of all your friends, and more importantly, the boys in your class. This sets the idea that fitness and activity in a male-dominated environment can be quite intimidating for women. But exercise and activity doesn't have to be this way. There is a reason why boutique gyms are popping up everywhere and becoming more and more successful. Women thrive in a group environment that provides support that sets them up for success.

Now we have so many different forms and levels of activity to suit your comfort level that help keep you healthy. Exercise is beneficial for your health, and can start at any level. Going from being on the couch to champion level is possible and can be done, but most available programs are developed for men to be most successful. A big component of getting to the next level of your fitness is pushing yourself during your workout, but more often, women are pushing themselves at the wrong times for their hormones, which leaves them worn out and increases their risk of injury. Specific types of exercise done at specific times of your cycle can much easier help achieve results from your workout. Recovery time is essential in a workout routine. Giving your body the proper time to rest and recuperate allows you to respect the time your body needs to bring the energy and intensity for your next workout and in life.

Where to Start?

Determine your current fitness level and frequency of exercise, and choose activities within that category:

- ✓ **Sedentary – walking, jogging, yoga, tabata**
- ✓ **Intermittent – weight lifting, HIIT, group classes**
- ✓ **Frequent – weight lifting, HIIT, advanced classes**

Now we have so many different forms and levels of activity to suit your comfort level and to keep you healthy.

Getting Started—Overall Approach to Exercise

- How to begin – Start with a small, achievable goal—something within reach that is going to get you going on the right foot. If it's just going for a walk every day for a week, great. If it's taking a cross-fit class, super. Search for something new. Or even go on Facebook and ask what new things your friends are into. When you have friends who love to workout, it's almost like a clique, and they will try to recruit you to their gym, so let them.

- Frequency/Recovery time – When getting started, it's very important to listen to your body. You may be sore, which is fine, but if you have hormonal issues that are preventing you from having a "normal" speed recovery, it's important you give your body the extra time needed to rest. Aim for doing some kind of activity that elevates your heart rate at least 3–4 times per week for at least 20 minutes will help you gain the most benefit.

- Intensity – vary intensity based on your ability. HIIT workouts are great for this. The first time you do it, push yourself hard for 1 of 6 sets. The second time, push yourself hard for 2 of 6 sets. This is a great way to see and feel that you are getting in shape, and stronger.

- Strength training – When we think of strength training, often we picture having to be in the gym lifting heavy

Foods That Aid in Recovery:

- Whey protein

- Branch chair amino acids (minimum of 6g)

- Fluids

- Minerals/electrolytes

- Glucose

weights. While this is definitely one variation, you can gain a lot of benefit from body weight exercises. Tons of valuable resources can be found online for at-home, body-weight workouts. If you are going to head to the gym, but have never lifted weights before, hire a trainer. They will help make sure you are doing appropriate exercises for your fitness level, and will monitor your form in order to avoid injury.

- Aerobic training – I am talking about cardio. Yes, I know a lot of mixed information on cardio is available. I am not recommending that you get on the elliptical for 2 hours. Aerobic training can be anything from taking a class, to boot camp, to short sprints. It's important to increase your heart rate to improve cardiovascular fitness. Start by giving yourself a measurement (time or distance) and try to increase it from there.

Every Little Bit Counts – When you look at your body and your health, it's important to consider the big picture. I encourage women to take a look at their day or week as a snapshot. Did you do more things, rather than not, that are getting you closer to your goal,? If yes, then that's great, *so keep it up*. It's not like you're going to do one workout and lose weight, or take this one little supplement and then lose weight. It is all cumulative. Every little thing you do counts, and it's either bringing you closer to your goal, or farther from it.

My client, Marissa, was looking for ways to start being active again, but didn't feel comfortable jumping into a gym setting quite yet. I asked her what she was currently doing, and she mentioned she really hadn't started anything because she didn't know where to start. I asked her how many days per week she could walk for 10 minutes? We set a goal for her to start walking 3 days per week for 10 minutes. After the first week she came back to me ecstatic that she had walked 5 days in a row for 15 minutes at a time. Marissa started feeling more confident, and had so much more energy just from her short walks. A couple weeks later she added in a short jog twice per week. Starting out slowly was exactly the push she needed to get moving again.

Make It a Habit – It takes 21 days to form a habit. I'm sure you've heard this before, but it's true. If you can keep something up for 21 days, you are much more likely to stick to it. So when it comes to implementing something new, or shifting your lifestyle, take small steps. Start out with the things you know you can stick to in order to make them "a habit," and continue to set a new benchmark from there. Pretty soon it will be like second nature.

> **"Don't expect to see positive changes in your life
> if you surround yourself with negative people."**
>
> **– Robert Tew, author**

Keep Fit Company – Your friends can make or break you, especially if you are trying to make positive changes for yourself. A good buddy will share healthy recipes with you, go for walks with you, and inquire about your progress. On the other hand, plenty of women who are working to improve themselves have friends that are a negative influence.

You may have heard the saying that you are most like the five people with whom you spend the most time. Many women socialize with a group of women. Throughout their relationship, they enjoyed a similar lifestyle. With time, if someone in the group decides to change, it throws everyone off. While many of the group's activities are centered around unhealthy choices—like eating too much of the wrong food, drinking too much, and not exercising—you can see how someone dedicated to a healthier lifestyle may throw a wrench in that.

What happens when that one person (hopefully you!) wants to try a healthier restaurant or a new activity rather than watching a movie while eating a tub of buttery popcorn? The friends start to notice, they may feel threatened, jealous, or disturbed by the change in the routines to which they have been accustomed. If you're the odd woman out who is trying to improve your life, and your friends are not supportive, the odds of success are against you.

Women need to realize that if they want to make a change, they either need to recruit their friends to join them, or they need find a new group that is supportive and will encourage the change. There's nothing like a group of women holding you accountable to showing up at the gym at 5:30 a.m. to get you out of bed and excited to work out. Or having a great accountability partner that will head straight to the gym from work with you so there are no excuses for not fitting it in.

Researchers have found that girls who work together in groups learn faster and score higher on tests than boys do. They also score higher compared to when they work individually. Women are very naturally inclined to communicate and gain support from each other that way. So, why not use the group mentality to tap into the resources you need to successfully meet your health goals?

**Find your community of supportive,
like-minded women and hang onto them.**

Exercise Strategies:

- **Resistance/Weight Training**

To keep the female body healthy, weight lifting is essential. I'm not saying you have to become a body builder, but doing at least light weights has shown to have tremendous benefit. Weight training increases your metabolism and switches on the fat-burning mode. It's true, you burn more calories for a longer period of time after weight lifting. If you aren't sure where to start with weight lifting, find a trainer. They can teach you how to perform certain key exercises, and will make sure your form is correct so you aren't placing unneeded stress on the body. In addition, when the bones are put under increased stress, like when weight lifting, they will maintain higher density by retaining more calcium in the bones. Studies have shown that women who lifted weights for one year had a significant increase in bone density in their spine and hips, which are the most common areas of the body where women lose bone density. This is important because hip fractures are the top reason that elderly people are admitted into nursing homes.

- **Interval Training**

  - Interval training is a type of exercise that involves a series of low-to-high intensity moves with a period of rest in between.
  - Interval training is another great way to help you burn more fat and then shock your body, keeping your metabolism running very high.
  - The beautiful thing about interval training is that your body does not get accustomed to it as long as you're changing exercises or changing the position that the body is in during the exercises. For instance, you will want to do some exercises upright and others

while lying down, thus changing the physical position of your body.

- If you are interval training and only doing sprints, your body is going to get accustomed to that. Instead of sprint, walk, sprint, walk, etc., try sprinting up the hill and then jogging down, sprint up a hill, jog down, and then do push-ups at the bottom of the hill.

• Exercise and Cortisol

Cortisol is often referred to as "the stress hormone." It is the hormone released by adrenal glands. When released during exercise, cortisol slows down your digestive system, increases your heart rate, decreases immune system function, stores fat, and breaks down muscle tissue. Great, right? I'm sure you are thinking, "But I thought exercising was good for me?"

When you are engaging in any type of exercise, you are putting stress on your body. Your body releases cortisol as its natural reaction. So what does all of this mean? Gone are the days of needing to spend 60 minutes on the elliptical. I actually advise against this. At the 30-minute mark of any kind of exercise, the body's natural function releases cortisol, having a negative reaction in the body in terms of getting through your workout routine in a beneficial way.

Cortisol will take protein and turn it into sugar, storing it as fat, which most likely results in the opposite of what you were initially working towards.

How can you avoid this? Keep your workouts shorter, and at the right intensity for where you are at in your cycle. If you are planning on working out for longer than 30 minutes, make sure you have a high-quality glucose source to push you through the second half. By shortening your workout, or adding in a glucose source at the 30-minute mark of your workout, can help you avoid derailing your goals.

Chapter 11:
Exercise and Mindset

Making positive changes in activity level can improve more than just your body, it has a huge impact on your mind. Countless studies show the positive effect that exercise has on the physical body. When you start exercising, your body releases endorphins that have been shown to boost mood and decrease physical pain in the body. Many studies link the benefit of exercise as helping those with depression and anxiety. Exercise recommendations are made for individuals with stress to counteract the negative side effects of stress and cortisol. Regular exercise has incredible health benefits on positive body image and self-esteem because as the physical body gets stronger, so does the projected self-image.

As we talked about in the nutrition chapter, it's important to set realistic goals for yourself. Take small steps. If you have never worked out before, expecting yourself to go to the gym five days per week is probably not realistic. But maybe parking at the back of the parking lot at work so you have to walk farther sounds more realistic.

Set yourself up for success.
Setting realistic goals is key to being successful.

Don't try to go from 0-100 overnight. That can be discouraging, and makes it easier to fail or give up. Consistently giving yourself new successful experiences allows you to be successful long term.

Most importantly, take action! You can set goals, and prepare, but until you take action, you aren't moving towards your goal. Daily, consistent action will get you there. As you build momentum, it will get easier, but you have to start somewhere. Make today the day.

Female Fat Solutions:
1. Set realistic, attainable goals,
2. Find something you ENJOY doing, and
3. Surround yourself with the right community.

Part 5:

Other Important Factors that
Impact Results

Chapter 12:
It Takes 90 Days to Change Your Hormones

Men start every day with roughly the same level of one primary hormone: testosterone. Testosterone levels are generally highest in the morning, and slowly decrease as the day goes on. Men can easily alter the testosterone levels in their body by adding certain substances or activities. Caffeine, alcohol, tobacco, watching or participating in sports, all can bump up testosterone levels. Yes, even watching a football team score a touchdown can increase hormone levels in men. Explains a lot, doesn't it?

In contrast, once a woman's system is out of whack it takes 90 days of consistent new behaviors and treatment to get her hormones back on track.

This is why any time a woman starts or stops hormone medications, such as birth control pills, she is told it takes three months for her body to fully adjust itself.

Now you can see why when a diet guru recommends a "21-day Diet" or cleansing program, a woman will probably be disappointed with the results. Those "quick fix" methods can throw off a woman's hormones, making her next cycle more symptomatic and increase stress in the body.

Worse yet, short programs will kick start weight loss, release some water weight and inflammation in the body, producing a great short-term result, but setting up a woman for long-term failure.

Chapter 13:
Visceral Fat – and Inflammation

Visceral fat is abdominal fat. When you burn it, you are burning burdensome fat away from your visceral organs, such as your liver, pancreas, and intestines, thus allowing those organs to function more optimally.

Excess visceral fat is linked to inflammatory diseases—which is why people who have other health conditions absolutely need a different plan in order to lose weight and keep it off. But women who are eager to burn off visceral fats get confused by the different exercise recommendations that they see on the Internet, hear from friends, or read in magazines. So much information tells people to do 60 minutes of cardio a day to decrease the visceral fat, but this is the opposite of what needs to happen.

The key to decreasing visceral fat is:

1. Increase your body's overall fat burning.

2. Practice fasting/cleansing days.

3. Exercise with interval training for 30 minutes or less, which will not increase your body's stress response.

Be sure not to confuse visceral fat with subcutaneous fat. Subcutaneous fat (under the skin) is found everywhere and is essential in the body. It responds to most diet changes (positive diet changes), but the visceral fat doesn't. Some people who look thin (may have lower subcutaneous fat) can still have an unhealthy amount of visceral body fat—and this can be life threatening, because it increases the incidence of dangerous diseases such as, heart disease, high blood pressure, stroke, high cholesterol, diabetes, breast cancer, and dementia.

Inflammation

Visceral body fat has a huge role in increasing the amount of inflammation in the body. The danger of inflammation is not talked about nearly enough. The inflammatory response is a natural immune response the body has to stressors. Inflammation has been tied to nearly every one of today's chronic diseases. What happens is that visceral fat releases a precursor to the inflammation chemical. Once this is triggered it, fuels the entire body process that exacerbates the early symptoms of disease. The good news is that one great way to start reducing subcutaneous and visceral body fat is *to eat good fats*.

Burning fat releases toxins, which is one of many important reasons why you need to drink a lot of water to help flush out the toxins. Don't be surprised if you are hungry because it is a normal response to your body burning fat.

Chapter 14:
PMS (Premenstrual Syndrome)

I had horrible periods, and was basically debilitated for a week. Cramping, bloating, fatigue, you name it, I experienced it. And it had been this way for years. I had tried anything and everything the doctors recommended with little-to-no relief. Dr. Beth immediately knew my hormones were having drastic shifts, and if we could level that out even a little bit, I would find some relief. I began on her plan of warming and cooling, and I stuck to it as closely as I could. After two months of going through the plan, I had experienced dramatic differences.

I seriously cannot believe how much better I am feeling. I got my period yesterday, and was surprised. Normally I know it's coming because I am down for the count for a couple days before. My cramping is way less, my period is more manageable, and I finally have the energy I needed to get through the day.

-Courtney, 34-year-old married mom of 2,

works as a Teacher.

The cramps, the bloating, the headaches, and other issues that come along with your menstrual cycle are not disorders. They are signals that your body chemistry is off and needs attention. It could be telling you something about *what, when, or how* you eat or exercise, or that your sleep habits need to change. It might be warning you about a medical condition that needs attention. No matter the cause, *PMS symptoms are not to be hidden, masked, tolerated, or ignored.*

Every cycle is different. It is a huge misconception to expect every period to be the same.

It is not inevitable that a woman will be bitchy, cranky, or crampy before or during her period. And, if you are cranky one month, it does not mean you will be cranky again the next. Your cycle is influenced by hormones, what you are fueling your body with, and your stress levels. All these variables can create many unpredictable conditions that affect the moving parts. But if you are chronically cranky, or regularly experiencing another symptom, perhaps an underlying issue needs to be investigated.

Most PMS and menstrual cycle symptoms can be alleviated or eliminated with a little applied knowledge. You can manage PMS many ways besides popping a Midol. Even better, when you learn to the read the symptoms and understand what they are trying to tell you, you can lose weight faster, improve your overall health and fitness, and feel better all month.

Common PMS Symptoms:

But imagine how life would be if you didn't have to feel that way, and didn't have to go through the same ordeal every month.

Premenstrual symptoms occur during the second half (progesterone phase) of your cycle. PMS affects each woman differently, and all women get different combinations of symptoms—from headaches, to cramps, to irritability. Well, you don't have to feel that way every month. Every symptom of premenstrual syndrome is a signal from your body telling you what it needs. Here we will review the nine most common symptoms, learn what they mean and how to manage, reduce, or eliminate each one by getting to the root cause. .

• **Mood Swings**

Ever get teary watching a diaper commercial? Or have you lost your temper because for the fortieth time you have to tell you kid to put her cereal bowl in the sink? Yeah, me too.

Before your period, your mood may be feisty, hyper-sensitized, and more stressed. Don't let it surprise you. Mood swings are an indication that a hormonal shift is taking place. More progesterone means more fatigue. More fatigue typically means more irritability. Your body is doing a lot in this phase, not only hormonally, but physically. Blood is being pulled away from your circulatory system and stored in a blood lining in the uterus. Vitamins, nutrients, even your vitality are being reallocated to support your menstrual cycle. When you are deprived of those things, *you are going to feel cranky.*

Plan for your potentially moody time by scheduling fun or relaxing activities and avoiding stressful situations.

Consider practicing yoga, carve out time to read, or lie down and rest. Make a point to watch an enjoyable movie or television show. Try your best to avoid situations that you know will stress you out—this may mean waiting a week to tackle a grueling project, avoiding your snarky sister-in-law, or scheduling your daughter's slumber party another time. It is important to take a multi-vitamin, fish oil, and vitamin C every day during this time.

- **Fatigue**

When your period draws near, sometimes you simply feel worn out. Normal routines are exhausting, and all you want to do is sit. It feels like it takes all of your energy—and then some—to complete even the most mundane tasks.

This is fatigue. Similar to moodiness, fatigue happens with the rising progesterone, which makes you tired. Plus, storing blood takes a lot of your energy, and nutrients. Give yourself extra rest and downtime in your schedule. Take vitamins regularly, along with other supplements including fish oil and iron.

- **Headaches**

I know a woman who suffers from a headache each Thursday before her period starts. She complains of pain in her left eye and ear, kind of like a sinus headache. Headaches like this, and those with other symptoms, typically arise because your hormones have suddenly shifted. Additionally, your body is not flushing toxins as quickly since your metabolism may not be running at top speed. If you're not exercising, problems may compound because you are not flushing out your lymphatic system by sweating.

Nutrient deficiencies can cause the headaches, as can blood-sugar issues or insulin sensitivity. Your body is using a lot of its stored energy, and it is burning more fats and wanting more sugar. You are burning energy at a higher rate, which may result in sharp blood-sugar drops causing you to feel hungry more quickly, especially if you do not get the right kind of fats earlier in the day.

To help prevent headaches, make sure to drink plenty of water, which is always a good practice.

Eat lots of healthy fats, which are unsaturated fats, included in foods like fish, avocados, almonds, walnuts, and flax, and do not allow yourself to get too hungry. I highly recommend adding in bulletproof coffee, and fat bombs.

I have some great recipes on my Facebook page (https://www.facebook.com/drbethwestie/).

Exercise will get you sweating and help you move toxins out of your cells.

There's much value in relaxing your muscle tissue. Relaxing muscle tissue will help take tension off of cramps, and helps flush toxins out of the body. That way, the progesterone hormone can move throughout the body without getting built up so much, or coming on so suddenly that it causes headaches. An Epsom salt bath is effective as well. Epsom salt is not actually salt, but a mineral compound of magnesium and sulfate, which are both easily absorbed through the skin. Magnesium has been proven to reduce inflammation and help muscle and nerve function. Sulfates help improve the absorption of nutrients, flush toxins, and help ease migraine headaches. And while your body is absorbing the healthful nutrients, the Epsom salts help pull out harmful toxins from your body.[xi]

Massage, including body brushing, a relaxation massage, and Swedish massage, promote detox drainage, as does a visit to the sauna or steam room. Another effective strategy against headaches is acupuncture.

• Bloating

While you are more prone to feeling irritable and sensitive, it's a cruel trick of nature that you might feel fat and uncomfortable at the same time. It's probably not true you've gained fat, but more likely you are just bloated.

During the second half of your cycle, you will possibly retain water, feeling full or swollen in your abdomen. Your digestive system slows down because your gallbladder is less active. Scar tissue developed from previous childbirths or abdominal surgery can make it worse. Any food you eat will move through your system slower than normal. If you eat foods that are difficult to digest, such as greasy, creamy, and fatty foods (unhealthy fats, such as saturated fat and trans fat), you are going to feel it. Eating the wrong foods causes inflammation because those foods are harder to break down. When inflammation takes hold in your lower abdomen, it can set off the cascade of other issues, such as swelling in the body, and feeling bloated like you are retaining water.

Help your system by eating fiber-rich foods and healthy fats.

This is a great time to eat beef and spicy foods to add heat to your system, which helps speed things along. Take extra fiber and extra probiotic, all of which helps your digestive tissue move things along.

Add a bit more salt to your diet. Western medicine advises against salt, citing fluid buildup and retention. In Chinese medicine, salt is the essence of life. They say you crave salt right before your period because your body needs it. You can help flush your lymph system with exercise, massage, Epsom salt baths or body brushing. Consume foods, such as lemon, grapefruit or oats, and drink more water.

- **Cramping**

Cramps are a gnawing pain felt in your lower abdomen and even your lower back. Though you will find various explanations for cramps, I blame the digestive system. During this time, you have a little bit more inflammation in your reproductive organs. Your uterus is swollen and filled with more blood. You are going to be more sensitive in the abdomen area anyway, and now you have this slower-moving matter moving through your digestive system. That's going to irritate some things, and you are going to feel it. If you have endured an abdominal surgery or given birth, often the scar tissue that builds up in your abdomen can affect your digestive system.

A hot compress is very soothing. It brings more blood to the area to help flush things out. It relaxes muscle tissue, and it helps your digestive system move faster while also physically bringing heat to the body in a phase where your body wants more heat, so it's all good things. Essential oils of lavender, peppermint and wintergreen are all good for relieving muscle tissue tension. I recommend either lemon water or putting essential oil lemon drops in your water, which helps detoxify and move things through the digestive system. Ginger is both very warming and an aid for digestion. Epsom salt baths and magnesium supplements help calm down the muscle tissue.

• Cravings – Heed True Cravings

We have all had those days when you have to muster the energy to get up off of the couch, wander to the kitchen, open the refrigerator, nothing; open the freezer, nothing. Your last hope is the pantry? Nothing. You are mindlessly wandering around, feeling sad, bored and plain blah, and you continue to search for something to eat and satisfy your craving. That, my friends, *is an emotional craving*.

Allow me to help you understand the difference between an emotional craving, and experiencing a true craving. Pay close attention and you'll realize that it is a different feeling. An example of a true craving is when you are about to get your period, and you have a strong desire for chocolate.

Once you become more in tune with your body and what it craves at certain times of your cycle you will eventually learn, what your body is truly craving as fuel.

Consider allowing yourself some of that food, but in moderation. As I have said before, you want to put quality foods into your body. So you're craving chocolate? Eat a nice piece a dark chocolate, not a cheap, waxy chocolate bar. You are craving something soft and creamy. Does is have to be a container of pudding? Or would a soft cheese be satisfying? Or you're craving salt? Okay. How about a piece of cheese? That will do your body more good than a half a canister of Pringles. Learn to be mindful about how you fulfill these cravings.

Be aware that some cravings are a sign of a deficiency, for instance, many people who crave chewing ice are anemic (same for those who eat dirt). People would say to a trainer friend of mine, "Well, I was really craving a donut." Her response is, "No. No! No part of your body ever says to itself, 'You know, I really needed a donut.'" It's important to make some distinctions here about what would be illegitimate. In your heart you know, yes, craving salt is legitimate. Craving Lucky Charms, not so much.

Trying to focus on work, but you can stop thinking about the bag of potato chips in the vending machine? We have all experienced them. A craving, an intense, urgent, or abnormal desire or longing for, you name it: chocolate, a steak, pizza, french fries, candy.

Cravings are normal. They are not weird. They are not wrong. They're signals from your body trying to tell you something. But be sure to satisfy your craving with health foods, not junk. Usually, premenstrual cravings are for extra sugar, fat, and salt. If you're not leveling out your blood sugars correctly first thing in the morning, by the afternoon, you are going to be craving those quick sugars to get your blood sugar going again, and so you feel you can return to acting like a normal person.

If you don't get enough healthy fat and salt early in the day, by afternoon you will be physically tired and mentally exhausted. What makes matters worse is that progesterone makes you even more tired.

I like to think I make an excellent premenstrual breakfast. I take greens—spinach, kale, chard, a tablespoon or two of coconut oil, put it in a pan and fry my greens a little bit. Then I add a couple of eggs. That way, I am getting my protein, my healthy fats, my good healthy greens, and my iron first thing in the morning.

• Back Pain

All the nerves that come from your spine go to your reproductive organs. It is not uncommon for women to say, "When my back hurts, I know I'm getting my period." That is because those nerves go to your organs, and your organs are slightly inflamed. The organs are filling with fluid, absorbing all those nutrients and vital essence. The nerves are irritated too because the nerve connects to the organ, so you feel it in your back.

Here is where treatments like a massage, a chiropractic adjustment, or acupuncture can help. Getting work done on your back can help your entire body.

Try using pain-relieving creams. I like a combination of heat and ice to alleviate the pain because it pumps fluid through the area. It can help alleviate both the back pain and with everything internally as well.

**When those nerves are happier,
everything inside will function better too.**

• **Diarrhea/Constipation or Both**

During the week before your period, your digestive system slows down. Eating things that irritate it will result in diarrhea, which is your body trying to flush out the irritants. For some women, constipation is a bigger problem. It is common to start out more constipated in the days leading up to the period, and then within a day or two of your period's arrival, you get a loose stool.

**Practicing self-care throughout the month
will lessen the severity and frequency of these digestive
issues.**

Consume probiotics. If your stools are loose, add in bananas and rice to your diet because they are more binding foods.

Add in digestive aids such as kombucha tea to ensure you have a healthy gut.

• Brain Fog

Let me tell you about brain fog. A friend in her early 30s arrived at the grocery store for her weekly shopping trip. List in hand, she combed through the aisles. Her cart was loaded full of groceries by the time she pushed it into the checkout stand. She paid and drove home. Once home, she popped open the trunk to start unloading. No groceries. She had apparently paid for them and promptly walked out of the store, leaving her bags behind. That's brain fog in action. (Don't worry for the checkers saved her bags for her, though they snickered a bit when she returned.)

What is commonly referred to as the "mommy brain," or "pregnancy brain," premenstrual brain fog makes it hard to concentrate, plus you'll find decision-making difficult, or you forget more than you usually do. Not a lot of research exists to indicate why this happens, but the likely culprit is the rapid hormonal shift and progesterone spike. You may not realize it until it is happening or, in some cases, not until the fog clears, and your wits have returned.

To help with this, be sure you are getting enough Vitamin D. Studies have shown that Vitamin D levels above 40 ng/mL (100 nmol/L) may reduce the risk of cognitive impairment.[xii] And be sure you're getting enough sleep.

Ashwaganda is an herb that also helps with overall mental clarity.

You know what makes everything better? Chocolate.

Seriously, it's good for your body, mind, and spirit. Chocolate's benefits include boosting energy levels, reducing blood pressure, and aiding in tissue healing. The chemical theobromine is responsible for chocolate being a vasodilator (meaning it increases blood flow). Raw cocoa and dark chocolate hold beneficial properties because the flavonoids degrade during cooking and alkalizing process. In addition, chocolate contains essential minerals that are not available from any other source. Studies have shown that short-term decreases in "bad" cholesterol levels happen with dark chocolate intake.

Chocolate that is at least 70 percent cacao contains essential minerals that are not available from any other source. Chocolate can improve exercise endurance, and is a great exercise recovery tool.

Benefits of Dark Chocolate:

- Weight loss

- Increased metabolism

- Faster tissue healing time

- More energy

- Decreased swelling

- Decreased blood pressure

- It is a diuretic

- It is a heart stimulant

- It is rich in antioxidants

- It relaxes smooth muscle

- It is an aphrodisiac.

To be clear, as tempting as that may sound, I am not suggesting you cuddle up with a book, blanket and a bag of Hershey's Kisses. Pick up a nice bar of dark chocolate, with at least 70 percent cacao, and nibble on a small piece of that bar once or twice a day as needed.

Chapter 15: Sleep— When You Snooze You Loose...More Weight

Sleep should not be a luxury. Sleep is a necessity, and a basic human need. I know women who feel guilty for sleeping in on the weekends or for catching a catnap during the afternoon. Don't, it's vital to your health.

According to the National Sleep Foundation (NSF), most people need seven to nine hours of sleep each night to function well the next day. In the foundation's *Women and Sleep* poll, researchers found that the average woman aged 30 to 60-years-old sleeps only six hours and 41 minutes during the workweek.[xiii] Another poll from the foundation found that women are more likely than men to have difficulty falling and staying asleep.[xiv]

Sleep deprivation causes increased accidents, poor concentration, a lowered immune system, and weight gain.

Evidence even suggests that there's a link between poor sleep and an increased risk of breast cancer.[xv] The foundation further acknowledged that women have sleep struggles due to menstrual cycles. "This is because of the changing levels of hormones that a woman experiences throughout the month and over her lifetime, like estrogen and progesterone, have an impact on sleep," according to NSF.[xvi]

Your body should drift through different stages of sleep, with two main types of sleep: 1) non-rapid eye movement sleep, known as quiet sleep, and 2) rapid eye movement sleep, known as active sleep or paradoxical sleep.[xvii]

Some people have trouble falling asleep, while others have problems staying asleep. Some people wake up in the middle of the night, always at the same time. If you ask a doctor about this, the recommended cure is, "Take an Ambian." But it is not like your body is naturally lacking Ambian, the prescribed sleep aid. Something else is going on.

Routines for Sleep

Not being able to fall asleep or stay asleep is often caused because people stay up too late and the body gets too fatigued. Then it is difficult to drop into a regular sleep rhythm. The top issue I encounter with clients is their inability to unwind at the end of the day. People watch the evening news, linger on Facebook or work right up until bedtime. Their minds get charged with negative thoughts, gossip, or problems at work. No wonder they toss and turn rather than falling into a deep, peaceful sleep.

The more regular you are with your sleep patterns, the easier it is when you are forced to adapt, like if you are traveling and staying in a different time zone.

Your body can jump on and off and get right back on its normal regular pattern much easier if you have regular pattern to begin with.

Then there are the instances when you have made all the right preparations for bed, but the kids squash your schedule. I put three kids to bed each night. At different times each one concocts a story about why she isn't asleep yet. She's scared, she's dying of thirst and won't last the night without water, or she's crying. No one knows why, but she's crying. You negotiate with them, tolerate the howling and end up frustrated and stressed out.

A pre-bedtime ritual is effective for all members of the family, like putting a couple of drops of lavender oil in the bath you take before bed, or even using it topically on your skin. I use it either on myself or on my kids to get them to slow down and unwind. It is relaxing and calming for them. Their bodies respond to the scent, and know that it is time for sleep, reducing bedtime nonsense.

Other bedtime rituals include reading either informative or positive information, relaxing, or meditating. Self-massage is effective, too. Use a cream or oil and rub it deep into your legs. Drink a calming tea, such as chamomile to slow down the body.

Routines for sleep can help everyone. Your body needs them, and responds better to them. Your body adapts to the rhythm of routine, which helps to regulate your hormones overall. And you get much improved sleep.

Although it may sound silly, think about animals. Dogs, for instance, do not understand daylight savings time, they start nudging your hand and acting restless when their bodies tell them it's time to get up. They get accustomed to a certain rhythm in the day.

Everybody responds better when following a routine.

Routines—Regularity in Your Schedule

Many women, especially moms, will look at this heading and laugh. "Regularity in my schedule? Huh? Is that even possible?!"

How can you have regularity in your sleep when you don't have regularity when you are awake? Women orchestrate everything, the kids, the husband, the holidays, and their own careers.

But creating a routine will serve as a panacea for not only your sleep, but will help your body rhythm, and your stress levels. And you're not the only one who benefits because children thrive on routines and schedules.

"A body without bones would be a limp impossible mess, so a day without steady routine would be disruptive and chaotic."
— **May Sarton, poet, author**

But creating a daily time structure is a challenge. Typically women are not caring only for themselves, and we are usually the ones who must adapt to whatever interruption or crisis that bubbles up. The Pew Research Center reports that 56 percent of working women say it is difficult for them to balance the responsibilities of their careers with the responsibilities of their family. In the same study, 40 percent of women say they always feel rushed.[xviii]

Meanwhile, scientists have found that routines help you and your family members feel safe and secure. They help everyone understand what is expected at certain times throughout the day. Structure in your life helps you to more easily organize your life and accomplish goals.

Dr. Heidi Grant Halvorson, a social psychologist and author, explained why routines can help reduce stress and increase success.

"Routines remove the need to deliberate over what you should do when (which takes time and energy), because once you've established a routine you've already made those decisions."[xix]

While I agree Dr. Grant Halvorson's research on routines, I know that *life happens,* and women constantly need to make adjustments. You are supposed to balance your work and balance your home life, but I don't think we ever do. A woman is either putting in more time at home or more time at work. And she often has to flip the switch more frequently than the man in her life because men seem to have more control over their balance.

A friend is a divorced single mother and a business owner. When her children were young, they lived with her every other week. During the weeks that she had the kids, her emphasis was on family. On the weeks her children spent with their dad, she worked tirelessly on her business, putting in 15–16 hour days. She was happy to do it, so she could spend more time enjoying her children the following week. Had she tried to keep everything "in balance" and divide her attention all the time, both her children and her business would have suffered. For her and most other women, it is a challenge, if not impossible, to have a "regular daily balance" of everything because that is simply not how our lives roll. The good news is that my friend created a routine that worked for her situation. Though she didn't follow the same routine day-to-day, she created routines for her career- focused week and routines for her family-focused week.

Even two-parent families face challenges adhering to routines.

Your son broke a wire on his braces, you are managing a special event at work, your car is in the shop, and suddenly everything you had planned is on the back burner, waiting for another time. You try to plan out your day, your week, your month, your everything, but life happens. And whether your husband is helpful or not, the responsibility to figure out how to get everything done, while still getting everyone fed and not forgetting a kid at soccer practice, typically lies with the woman in the family.

Life for a woman is a perpetual juggling act, and to survive, she learns to adapt to every situation. But she will be happier if she can establish some routines to help create a framework for accomplishing mundane tasks and achieving long-term goals. Although on some days, you'll have to scrap schedules and fight fires, a daily routine will help you on a very basic level.

Consider your eating routines. If you eat every two to three hours, and then suddenly go four hours without eating, your body will get hungry. You have trained yourself to follow a certain routine. Your body knows what to do. Even in the midst of a crisis, your body will signal for you to eat because that is your routine. That is a good thing.

Although the day's events didn't go as planned, at least your routine helped you remember to take care of your own basic needs.

Chapter 16: Stress— *It's Time for Stress to Take a Hike*

As many women do, I felt like I was doing all the right things. Eating right, exercising when I could, and overall juggling life as a mom and businesswoman. However, I didn't get the weight loss results I was seeking, and couldn't figure out why. A lot of the suggestions Dr. Beth made me resonated with me, and I was doing most of it. But one piece was missing. When we dove into the topic of stress, I said that I didn't really feel "stressed." I had the typical daily stuff every mom and career woman deals with. But, when we dug a little deeper, we discovered a couple things here and there continued to trigger the stress response that I was not even aware of. Once we determined what those things were, we set up a strategy to help me combat those situations, and decrease the stress response in her body.

Sure enough four weeks in, I was starting to notice the weight come off! After eight weeks of working with Dr. Beth, I was down 12 pounds, 17 inches, and felt like I had more energy than ever before.

– Holly, 37 year old married mom of 3, works as a Marketing Director for a corporate company.

Let's pause here for a reminder about keeping it real. Life is real. Sickness, broken cars, and forgetful children are real as are schedules that are blown to pieces. By trying to reach these unrealistic expectations that are more conducive to a man's world, women begin to feel inadequate, "less than," and it causes them stress.

As said earlier, any of the recommendations for weight loss are more realistic for men than women—from consistent workouts to consistent eating throughout the month. Women take these recommendations to hear, like what they "should" do to be successful. They assume other women are experiencing "success" by living by these recommendations, and meeting their goals.

But everyone will have bad days and "setbacks," and the best intentions that go awry. Try not to let it stress you out because when you are stressed, no matter what the cause, your body secretes the hormone cortisol. While cortisol is necessary for survival, too much cortisol is a bad thing. It causes an inflammatory response in your body. It can affect your immune system, digestive system, your heart, your skin, and reproductive system.

Do not underestimate the effects of stress for it can be a serious threat to your health.

A University of Kentucky study found that dieters who learned stress-management tactics were more successful at losing weight than dieters who didn't.

The connection between reducing stress and losing weight could be that it helps cut back on stress-related binge eating. The journal *Psychoneuroendocrinology* found that women who were constantly stressed out metabolized fat and sugar differently than those who weren't anxiety-ridden. [xx]

Another study, released by the British Nutrition Foundation, found that women who are stressed tend to make poor food choices that cause them to gain weight. Talk about adding insult to injury! C.J. Roberts, from the Institute of Psychiatry at King's College in London, found an increase in cortisol secretion during a period of chronic stress to be strongly correlated with changes in food choice and increased calories, as well as an increase in intake of saturated fatty acids. This resulted in an increase in bodyweight. They also found that women with a body mass index (BMI) on the higher side of "healthy," who experienced a significant increase in cortisol secretion under chronic stress, were more vulnerable to increases in bodyweight than women with lower BMIs. [xxi]

So, if you're already a bit overweight, and you get stressed and eat unhealthy foods, you are more likely to gain weight than a thin person who does the same thing.

No one ever said your body chemistry *was fair*.

Here we will focus on physical stress, which can happen if you exercise too much or the wrong way.

An example of physical stress is running on a treadmill for an hour every day. The result: it increases your physical cortisol in a way that is not good. After 30 minutes of activity, your cortisol levels are going to rise because your body is the fight-or-flight response.

- If you are trying to get your metabolism working properly, limit

Signs You Might Be Stressed: [22]

- **Frequent headaches, jaw clenching or pain.**
- **Gritting or grinding your teeth.**
- **Stuttering or stammering.**
- **Tremors, trembling of lips or hands.**
- **Neck ache, back pain, muscle spasms.**
- **Light headedness or faintness or dizziness.**
- **Ringing, buzzing or popping sounds.**
- **Frequent sweating or being flushed**
- **Cold or sweaty hands or feet.**
- **Dry mouth or problems swallowing.**

exercise to a maximum of 30 minutes, unless you already exercise regularly or you are an athlete. For instance, I have been a high-level athlete my whole life, so my body is accustomed to handling that higher level of cortisol.

If a person is already under a lot of stress at home or at work, an illness or a life change, then limit exercise to 15 or 20 minutes.

For example, imagine a fit, active person who lifts weights and does cardio as part of her normal routine; then her mother dies. Now she is under a completely different level of stress that is psychological and can be long-term. Although that stress is emotional rather than physical, your body does not differentiate between the two. Your system has still more cortisol, resulting in more stress overall. Yes, many people recommend exercise as a way to improve your mood. It certainly will boost endorphins, but exercise adds physical stress to a body that is already experiencing emotional stress. When these life events happen, I recommend shorter bouts of exercise that will get the endorphins flowing without completely taxing your body.

What works for you and what stresses your body will be entirely different than what works for your friend or sister-in-law. It is highly individual.

- ✓ Do you already have an exercise routine?

- ✓ Are you on your feet all day, and constantly moving?

- ✓ Are you mostly sedentary?

Cortisol

Increased Cortisol Levels can:

- **Weaken immune system.**
- **Decrease bone formation.**
- **Inhibit collagen—especially in skin, and it can take 40 percent longer to heal wounds.**
- **Decrease metabolism.**

Getting Back on Track – You Fell Off the Wagon, Now What?

What do you do when inevitably you get off track?

I planned to get up at 5:00 a.m. to get to the gym and back before my kids wake up around 6:30 when I have to make breakfast, lunches, and get them out the door for school an hour later. At 3 in the morning, my youngest is screaming at the top of her lungs because she has a bloody nose. By time I clean her up and get her back to bed, it's 3:45. I shut my eyes for what feels like 2 minutes when my oldest comes in telling me he's throwing up. I know my plan for the morning is completely shot. Sound familiar? Even if I can't get my entire workout in, I will make time to do something. Maybe it's a quick HIIT workout, or a run. Regardless, don't allow those life things that are bound to happen, derail you completely.

Now it's your kid's birthday weekend. We all do our best to make the "right" choices, but it's ridiculous to expect there will be no temptations. More than likely your normal routine is going to be out the window. There will be cake, and if you are like me, there will be wine. I believe you should have that piece of cake, and that glass of wine. That's life, and you should enjoy it. However, eating the entire cake, or drinking two bottles of wine, is a different story. If you allow yourself to have indulges here and there, you are much less likely to devour the entire cake. Promise yourself that you will get right *back on track tomorrow.* Don't let one "bad" food choice end up being a week of "bad" meals.

Chapter 17:
Value of Herbs and Supplements to Your Body's Overall Health

I could write an entire book on the health benefits of nutrition supplements and herbs. But for now, I want to at least offer you a concise rundown on some of my favorites. When you are perusing the store shelves, always select quality products. Read the labels to make sure you are getting the most quality for your money. When considering your dosage, use the label on the bottle as a basic reference, knowing however that you may need more of the supplement. The amount a person needs varies. It is not an exact science, but a trial-and-error system. You need to experiment to make sure you are getting enough of what you need. Some people will take the recommended daily dosage, and still be deficient. For some of the nutrients you can get a blood test to assess what your levels are. Be sure to buy from companies that have their product tested by an independent third party.

- **Multi-vitamin** – Select an option that is whole-food based, meaning they essentially take tons of organic broccoli, kale, and other vegetables, making them into a powder and cramming it in a capsule.

- **Fish oil** – I recommend two capsules of the fish oil daily. It provides extra benefits in terms of omega fatty acids, and it is anti-inflammatory. Make sure you choose a fish oil that is from a clean source, like fresh, wild salmon. The capsules should not smell fishy.

- **Vitamin D** – Your primary source of vitamin D is from sunshine. But some people do not make time for that, or may need more. For them, I recommend Vitamin D supplements. You can find the vitamin in capsule form or liquid form.

- **Probiotic** – Taking a probiotic is fantastic for digestion. It helps break down foods, improves your body's absorption of nutrients, and is better for your immune health. Make sure to select a quality project—my favorite is Innate Choice. Remember, this product must be refrigerated.

- **Herbs – Incorporate These Herbs into Your Diet:**
  o Holy basil: helps with adrenal fatigue, hypothyroidism, blood sugar, and acne, as well as worry and nervousness
  o Ginsing: provides an energy boost, lower blood sugar and cholesterol, reduces stress, and promotes relaxation
  o Ashwaghanda: helps with
    1) stress and cortisol levels,
    2) the endocrine system (estrogen, progesterone, thyroid),

3) stamina and endurance, blood sugar, and adrenals, and

4) fertility

- o Eluthro (Siberian Ginsing): boosts energy, brain function, stamina, recovery, and immune system, and also decreases inflammation
- o Tumeric: anti-inflammatory, decrease stomach issues, natural detoxifier, antioxidant, brain boosting. Helps with worry and nervousness.
- o Wolf berry (Goji Berry): improves eye sight, immune function, antioxidant, liver detoxification, boosts kidney function, improves skin health and helps with liver health

Hormone Replacement

Women have managed to get their monthly periods, have one for decades, and then go through menopause without drugs up until the 1970s, which is when hormone replacement therapy started. Now, it is like we think we cannot survive without these drugs. The expectation is that when women enter this stage of life, they should go on hormone replacement therapy. Your body is going through a difference phase at this time, and it needs different support. So rather than masking that with drugs, we need to give our body what it needs.

One patient was getting hot flashes. She started taking progesterone supplements. The hot flashes stopped for a while, but started up again. She decided to stop taking the supplements, and cut way back on her sugar and alcohol. Guess what? She hasn't had a hot flash in months. I believe that many menopausal symptoms can be addressed by changing your diet and through self-care, like getting more sleep.

Many health risks are associated with hormone replacement therapy, like heart disease and stroke.

My problem with hormone replacement therapy is that it is *bioidentical,* meaning that it is not naturally derived so it will not be a close match to what your body produces on its own. Hormone replacement therapy wasn't even designed to be used for a typical menopause situation. It is designed for specific situations, for example, a woman who needs an emergency hysterectomy for some reason. She will have some sudden hormone shifts at that point, so to be thrown into full-blown menopause is a lot for the body to handle. It's designed for a short-term transition, but then a woman should wean herself off it.

You need to allow your body to go through this natural phase of womanhood. Listen to what your body needs, and then respond accordingly. A medical doctor may readily offer you hormone therapy to make you more comfortable during the transition. But, to be honest, I have a problem with people who think that they should simply float through life, and never feel uncomfortable. Feeling discomfort is your body's way of saying that you need to make some changes. The body needs different care throughout its different stages.

Babies, toddlers, and kids all need naps in the afternoon. Their bodies need more sleep, and their body physically needs something different. It's a different phase and change of life.

Through menopause and other stages of life, you have to change how you eat, change your sleep, and change your exercise routine. Change how you take care of yourself so you will feel better while you go through this phase of life. However, our society doesn't think that way. What do we do instead? We mask our symptoms with hormone replacement therapy, and women have ended up with a higher risk of stroke, heart disease, and cancer.

Female Fat Solutions

1. Identifying key PMS symptoms and their real meaning is the best starting point for understanding the underlying issue.

2. Getting into a routine is key to being successful.

3. Finding a solution that works for you to combat stress is necessary to help you reach your goals.

Videos:

✓ The Low Down on Stress:

✓ https://www.youtube.com/watch?v=MVpZOC6R3ro

✓ How can nutrition help with PMS symptoms? https://www.youtube.com/watch?v=mZyHrp--Lrc

Part 6:

The Seven Bodies of Eve

The female body goes through many changes throughout a lifetime. Each version of "Eve" requires different care, and different strategies for fat loss. In this chapter, I will provide an overview of the "seven bodies of Eve" that a woman may experience in her lifetime. The age ranges I list here are based on averages, so don't be alarmed if you went through a phase at a different age. Not all women experience all seven bodies, so as you read, simply focus on the ones that are relevant to you or someone you care for.

For each "body" we will look at five key distinctions:
1.   Hormonal status
2.   Nutritional considerations
3.   Physical and mental energy
4.   Tolerance for exercise and recovery
5.   Fat-loss strategies

Chapter 18:
Pre-Puberty (ages 7–11)

Hormonal status:

My seven-year-old daughter and four of her friends had been running around the house playing, and said they were thirsty. "What do you want to drink?" I'd asked. I heard several requests for water, which is normally my daughter'sfavorite, so I poured five glasses. When I handed my daughter's glass to her, I was surprised to get this response as she stood in the kitchen and sobbed. "No! I didn't want a glass of water!"

I went through my mental checklist. Is she getting along with her friends? Check. Did she get enough sleep? Check. Did she eat a good breakfast? Check. Is she in a growth spurt? Nope.

If I didn't know better, I might have thought she was just being a snotty brat. But even a little shift in hormones is a lot for a tiny body to process, and when a girl is that young, she has no experience navigating the feelings that a little burst of estrogen can induce.

Between the ages of seven and 11, most girls begin to experience their first spikes in estrogen. It's a precursor to starting her menstrual cycle. Usually the only symptom is bizarre and sudden shifts in mood. While these episodes typically don't last long, they aren't resolved as quickly when a child is tired or hungry.

Speaking calmly, hugs, personal touch for at least 30 seconds, will help her feel better, and it releases *oxytocin*, the hormone that makes us feel bonded and loved.

This is the first point where the female body begins to need different nutrients than the male. Girls' bodies start to change with hormonal shifts, and as a result, you may notice moodiness along with physical changes and some changes in energy levels. The changes are unpredictable. Some girls will start showing signs of puberty, regress, and then start again. Others will start, stall at one stage for a while, and then continue on until puberty hits and the body (eventually) establishes a regular cycle.

If you have a daughter, realize any time she is experiencing those changes, you can start tracking her hormonal cycle simply by observing her behavior. Though your data may not be exact, you can glean information that can help you be supportive emotionally as well as provide her optimal nutrition throughout the month.

As you learn how to work with your own body, be sure to pass this along to your daughters or any young girl in your care.

• **Nutritional considerations** – Follow standard guidelines for basic nutrition. You are helping your daughter to establish healthy foundations. Remember to include foods that contain healthy nutrients, such as calcium, which helps reduce the chance that she'll develop osteoporosis later in life.

- **Physical and mental energy** – Pre-adolescent girls are naturally at peak energy levels during this phase as their bodies are going through their last big growth push. Make sure girls this age get enough rest. To help optimize her chances of getting good rest, cut off her use of electronics an hour before bed. A girl can massage a couple of drops of peppermint oil or lavender oil into her skin to help her unwind at night.

- **Exercise** – This is a great age to give your child options of where to get involved. Explore multiple things. The benefit of experimenting with multiple sports during this time gets nerves and muscles firing in multiple ways: yoga, hiking, soccer, softball, gymnastics, dance, short-distance running. Don't worry about going for high-level performance. It's more about trying lots of activities and developing strength, coordination, and endurance to apply to many forms of athletics. As a rule, before the age of 13, lifting weights is not recommended. The body isn't proportioned yet, so the structure for proper weight lifting mechanics isn't in place.

- **Fat-loss strategies** – If the young woman in your life is eating too much junk food, or experiencing too much weight gain, a safe, healthy way to get a girl's system back on track is to do a light carb cycle. I'm not recommending anything dramatic because we're talking about a young person who is growing. Consider a 150-gram carbohydrate day, followed by 100-gram day and then a 75-gram day. That would easily get her body's metabolism revved, help her burn carbs, and get her weight under control.

In Chapter 6 under Nutrition, I wrote more on carb cycling and how to employ it in your nutritional program.

Chapter 19:
Adolescent (About Ages 12-21)

• **Hormonal status** – Menstrual cycles typically begin in this stage. With cramps, mood swings, energy shifts, and sometimes heavy bleeding, these girls are officially transitioning into young women. It is the time in life when many young women chose to go on birth control pills for a variety of reasons, from managing difficult menstrual cycles to preventing pregnancy. A lot of girls this age are prescribed birth control pills to regulate their menstrual cycle. If you are caring for a female this age, you will be doing her (and yourself) a favor if you share with her what you learn in this book in order to help her figure out how to use diet and exercise to train her body to regulate her cycle naturally. Help her with strategies you will learn in this book, and you will both be happier.

• **Nutritional considerations** – It is true for all women, at whatever age, that if they eat the right foods at the right time, they're going to feel better. When your body has the nutrients it needs, it functions at its best. Adolescence is a growth-spurt phase, and during those times, girls should be especially mindful about eating a healthy, balanced diet, and adding a little more protein (13 to 20 grams extra protein during growth spurts). Be sure she gets enough iron. If she is anemic, doesn't have enough iron, her body won't be able to utilize the protein it needs to grow new muscle tissue. The adolescent female can make a lot more "mistakes" with nutrition without right away seeing the impact on her body. However, this is when habits are established. As the body ages, it doesn't process foods the same way, and if eating junk is the norm, obesity and other health issues are more likely to occur.

• **Physical and mental energy** – Adolescents need more rest than any other time in life except when they were toddlers. They need a lot of energy for growth spurts, and sleep is a key factor in making sure they have that energy. Ideally, adolescents should get 12 hours of sleep a night, but as you probably know from your own experience, few adolescents get anywhere near this. Lack of sleep affects attitude, mood, growth, mental acuity, focus, concentration, and a myriad of other aspects of the adolescent's life.

• **Tolerance for exercise and recovery** – The good news is that adolescence is one of the easiest times to exercise and recover quickly. This is a great age to introduce weight lifting. It is easier to build muscle during this phase. Studies have shown that girls who do weight training, and take calcium in their teen years, retain more bone strength throughout their lifetimes than girls who don't. [xxii] This can help ward off osteoporosis. Note: If a girl is experiencing a growth spurt, she will need more than the usual time to recover after exercise.

• **Fat-loss strategies** – I worked with a mother and daughter for several years—and both were overweight. Mom was in her 50s. The daughter, 16, started asking me questions, "What's better for you, kale or spinach?"

"They're both good," I answered. Not understanding that underneath her questions was an agenda.

She had been reading in a woman's magazine about stars and their diets. I explained that actresses do all kinds of nutty diets to slim down for a movie role—and the stuff you're reading is not true. Fitness models don't always have six-pack abs all the time. They do extreme diets to lean down before a shoot.

We then learned that the daughter had taken cash that her mom had given her, got a Visa gift card, and used it online to buy diet pills she had shipped to the house.

Mom was heartbroken. I sat down with the daughter and explained healthy eating and healthy timing of eating, like fats and protein in the morning, carb cycling, etc.

Moving into adult world, lots of stress. The No. 1 fear for females around losing weight is that friends will no longer accept her, which is especially difficult for an adolescent where "friends are your life" at this stage.

Body image issues normally begin in this stage, and can impact any type of girl.

Fat loss during this age is recommended only if a physician suggests that the girl needs to lose weight. I don't want to encourage any girl or young woman of normal body weight who's in the "I'm fat," frame of mind, to obsess over weight loss. However, if a doctor expresses some serious concerns, such as poor insulin sensitivity or a Type 2 Diabetes diagnosis, a young woman can cycle carbs. This method will kick her metabolism into gear and teach her to how to use good to get results from her body quickly.

Chapter 20:
Competitive Athlete (All Ages)

A woman who sweats it out at least four times a week is considered a competitive athlete. She's working her body, building muscle, strengthening her cardiovascular system, and getting her heart rate up on a consistent basis.

Hormonal status – Female athletes tend to be lean and fit, especially highly competitive or elite-level athletes who participate in distance running, gymnastics, swimming, and dancing. These gals may start missing their periods, which is technically called *amenorrhea*. The missed periods are a result of the combination of intense physical activity and a low percentage of body fat. Amenorrhea is most likely to happen when a female is in a phase of intense training for a big event. Besides the physical activity and low body fat, the other variable that can be a factor *is stress.*

Stress impacts the hormones. When a person trains intensely, the body's level of cortisol increases. Factor in a low percentage of body fat, along with constantly exerting large amounts of effort and energy, and that combination kills her period. If the body was only experiencing the stress, a female may miss a period or two. But when you combine all three of those factors, her period may disappear for a while.

Amenorrhea can impact a woman's ability to follow this program because if her body is constantly under stress, she will have a difficult time maintaining a basic energy level that allows her to sustain her workouts and basic routines. What can make matters worse is if she is also limiting calorie intake. For instance, a young woman who is a cheerleader, wearing a little skirt all the time, may worry about her physical appearance, and, as a result, be very rigid on her calories and nutrient intake. Not only can this cause amenorrhea, but this kind of diet, along with the intense exercise and low percentage of body fat, can impact her overall health. A woman's peak bone density is built from ages 18 to 25. Denying the body what it needs during that phase can later result in an increased risk of complications such as broken bones, longer healing times, and osteoporosis.

If your body is under so much stress that your period stops, that is a warning sign saying, "Hey, this is a big deal. I am not getting what I need."

• **Nutritional considerations** – Athletes, and especially girls who are still growing, need more calories. Their bodies are under stress and burn through nutrients at a faster pace. Although culture has taught us that eating "fat" is bad, it is not true. People need fat. It provides a high concentrated form of energy, and it helps your body absorb, transport and store vitamins and nutrients.

Athletes should eat well before, during, *and* after competition. The body needs nutrients both for the competition and afterwards, so it can recover faster.

Most athletes eat well in the days before and the day of a competition, but after the finale, they go and celebrate with pizza. The post-competition meal should always be a healthy one to help the body recover, so you don't feel sluggish the next day. Simply grilling chicken breast and vegetables on the grill is a much healthier option. You've got to rebuild the body with those fuels correctly.

• **Physical and mental recovery** – Recovery days after a competition are important to a female athlete's overall wellbeing. A diligent recovery effort will affect the body's ability to bounce back and for the energy it will need for the next competition.

Generally, athletes underestimate the importance of recovery. They think, "Oh well, I go out and play for two hours a day every day, and I'll participate in this huge tournament on the weekend." Then they wonder, "Why is my body breaking down? Why am I getting injured? Why is my shoulder so sore and feel like it's wearing out?"

Most athletic injuries are caused by overuse. But most of these injuries can be prevented by properly fueling the body, and by getting adequate rest.

Imagine a high school distance runner. She would be training more than most people do. During periods of intense training or competition, like her high school season, the track meets come so frequently, she is going to need support from a parent to teach her how to help her body recover. Even a 30-minute massage once per week would help her body recover faster, repair itself, and replenish. Other effective techniques include acupuncture, physical therapy, or visiting a chiropractor. Give her ice packs, vitamins, and supplements.

For a while I helped with an elite girls' volleyball team. These girls and their mothers talked about using personal trainers and getting massages. It was normal for them. Some even had a massage therapist come to their homes. They knew if they wanted to make it to the next level, to play in college or beyond, taking care of their bodies was going to make a positive impact on their performance level.

Ways to help the body recover:

- Ice

- Massage

- Vitamins and supplements

- Physical therapy Chiropractic treatment

• **Tolerance for exercise and recovery** – An athlete's body functions at a high level. Because of this, athletes have a higher tolerance for the stress hormone, cortisol. Athletes can burn through the cortisol, and their body system is strong enough to handle it. Over time, that cortisol level is like the strengthening part of their program—strengthening them instead of breaking them down.

- **Fat-loss strategies** – Sometimes gymnasts, runners, swimmers, or other athletes want to lean out and decrease body fat percentage. In the midst of a competitive season, *do not attempt to lose body fat*. A more appropriate time to lean out is during pre-season or training season. But even then, your body still needs fuel, so the best way to achieve that lean body is through carb cycling. But carb cycling would look a bit different for an athlete. Rather than dipping down to 50 grams of carbs for a low day, their low day would range between 100–225 grams of carbs.

Chapter 21:
Pregnancy (Ages 16-45)

• **Hormonal status** – During pregnancy, women experience a sudden bump in progesterone and an increase in the growth hormone. Depending on the person, you can experience a wide variety of symptoms from those hormone shifts. Some women notice the growth hormone part of it, and feel energetic. This growth hormone makes a woman feel great and glowing. For other women, the overriding feeling may be one of total fatigue and struggle—like me, for example. I felt like my body was going haywire.

During the first trimester of pregnancy, all the important stuff is being formed, like the baby's brain, spinal cord, heart, lungs, etc. That's why pregnancy takes the most of out of our energy levels during the first three months. Fortunately, women tend to feel better during the second trimester because her body adapts to the surge in hormones related to pregnancy.

• **Nutritional considerations** – When a woman is pregnant, she needs to adjust her nutrition. In the first trimester, she needs to double up on her intake of fish oil to get enough omegas for the baby's brain development. I often recommend either doubling up or taking 1.5 times the amount of a multi-vitamin. Having extra nutrients in the body is not going to hurt anything, and your body will flush out whatever you don't need.

One of my daughters was born two months premature. But she weighed five pounds and was very healthy. She had no physical problems at all, no asthma, no other breathing problems even though she was born before her lungs were supposed to be developed, but I had taken a ton of vitamins. People could not believe she was a preemie. That is one of the reasons I am such a strong advocate for vitamins as part of your overall good health.

- **Physical and mental energy** – The sudden shift in hormones with an increase in progesterone can lead a lot of women to feel a radical dip in energy level, and many report "pregnant brain" as a pervasive fogginess, especially throughout the first trimester. By the second trimester, many women feel more of the affects of the growth hormones instead. Human Growth Hormone (HGH) can make a woman feel energized, and can induce that "glowing" feeling and an overall sense of contentment and wellbeing.

- **Tolerance for exercise and recovery** – If you exercised regularly before you became pregnant, it is safe to keep your routine during pregnancy. For example, if you ran five miles a day before, it is safe to run five miles while you are pregnant because your body is used to it. But if you have not been exercising, I recommend walking about 20 minutes a day and practicing pregnancy yoga. It is amazing the number of health benefits 20 minutes of walking can bring. But always remember to use common sense. A pregnant body is a strained body. Respect your body's signals and don't overstrain.

• **Fat-loss strategies** – Pregnancy *is not* the time to lose weight. Do not try any crazy diets. Focus on eating healthy foods that are loaded with vitamins and nutrients. The baby needs all those things, plus fats. And a pregnant woman needs it all, too. Healthy foods will help keep energy levels up, the immune system functioning well, and all systems running on target.

Chapter 22:
Postpartum Recovery and
Beyond (Ages 16–45)

- **Hormonal status** – prolactin, oxytocin, progesterone drops, 4–6 weeks to start period again or longer, may not have cycle for a while. After 4–6 weeks, start eating for your cycle again. Can take nine months to a year for pregnancy hormones to be out of the body.

- **Nutritional considerations** – needs extra calories to produce milk, higher body fat than usual to keep producing milk. Eat healthy fats because that is a big help in cutting down body fat when you're nursing. I suggest adding 3 extra tablespoons of coconut oil in the morning, along with your supplement vitamins and minerals.

- **Physical and mental energy** – first month, you don't know your head from your toes. Not sleeping well. Nursing — baby takes energy there, too. Ideally, when the baby sleeps, you should also sleep, for at least three months after giving birth.

- **Tolerance for exercise and recovery** – uterus is shrinking, ligaments are loose, energy is lower, usually. Aside from taking light walks, wait 2–3 months (2 months for vaginal birth, 3 months if Caesarian) before you start to do more intense exercise. As long as you're nursing, your tolerance and recovery is going to be limited.

- **Fat-loss strategies** – eating more healthy fats (in the morning) will help you lose fat. And carb cycling will rev up your metabolism. NO FASTING DAYS.

Chapter 23:
Perimenopause (Ages 40–60)

Normally when I go on vacation, I know I'll gain five pounds because I eat crap and drink wine for a week, but this time I gained ten pounds, and it's not coming off even though I am exercising. What the heck?"

I had done a lot of low-carb, no-carb stuff long term over six months to a year, which slows a woman's metabolism, affects the nervous system and endocrine system. I know the body is not designed for extreme low-carb dieting, and it creates a yo-yo dieting effect. Eventually, it becomes nearly impossible to lose weight.

Like a lot of women in this age range, I was 20 pounds over where I wanted to be, but I allowed myself to only think about losing 10 — because I had experienced so much discouragement while trying multiple diets and not seeing results.

Dr. Beth coached me to do a carb cycle. It is vital in this situation to be on point with grams of carb every day for the duration of the period that it takes to reset your metabolism, usually one to three months.

The first few weeks, I didn't lose any weight. In fact, I put on a couple pounds. Following the plan, I was able to drop the 10 pounds of vacation weight plus an additional 3 pounds for a total weight loss of 13 pounds. And I was so surprised. With the encouragement I felt from achieving my goal so easily, next, I wanted to take it farther, so Dr. Beth had me cycle in a few fasting days.

Last time I checked in, I had dropped 18 pounds and was cruising toward my true goal of losing 20 pounds.

– Cathy, 48-year-old, married mom of 2, works as an Radiologist.

• **Hormonal status –** This is what I call the "winding-down" period for the menstrual cycle. When you are an adolescent, it takes time for your period to regulate. A young woman may have a period; then go months without one. Or she may only experience spotting for a few months.

Just as it takes time for the menstrual cycle to start and become regular, it can take a while for menstruation to stop. Some women might say, "Yup, one day my period started, and it has been regular from that day on. Then it stopped, and that was it." But that's not how it goes for most women. During this winding-down phase, women are experiencing perimenopause. Estrogen and progesterone hormone levels are dropping. Progesterone goes first; then estrogen. Progesterone is mainly produced by the ovaries, although smaller amounts are produced by the nerves and fat tissue in your brain and your adrenal glands. During perimenopause, the ovaries basically become dormant, so the amount of progesterone produced goes way down.

You may find yourself saying:

- "I can't sleep anymore."
- "I'm getting hot flashes."

– "I don't know my body anymore."

If women are experiencing so much discomfort that it is interrupting their lives, and they have tried the carb cycling, exercise and the natural remedies, hormone replacement therapy may be a good option. But before you ask for a prescription, try "cleaner eating" first. One of my clients was having intense hot flashes throughout the day and night. They interrupted her sleep, and every day when she got dressed, it was no more than five minutes after she was out of the shower when a hot flash would leave her drenched in sweat. Instead of taking progesterone, she reduced her consumption of sugar and alcohol from having a little treat and a glass of wine each day to only indulging once or twice a week—and her hot flashes vanished.

• **Nutritional considerations** – Moderation is the key when it comes to nutrition. At this stage of your life, you may need to experiment with foods that help you manage the ups-and-downs of perimenopause. For example, some women feel better if they reduce alcohol or cut caffeine. But in all likelihood, the dietary changes a woman needs to make at this point are temporary. It may be for a couple of months, or for a couple of years.

In general, I recommend eating cooling foods to regulate your cycle and help you feel more comfortable. *Always avoid inflammatory foods, such as sugar, dairy, red meat, gluten, and alcohol.* These modifications do not need to be permanent, but adjusting the food you eat to be in harmony with what your body is experiencing, results in a more comfortable, energetic, happier you.

• **Physical and Mental Energy** – Nutrition is a dominant player when it comes to your physical and mental energy. Of course, exercise is fantastic, as it's good for flushing the hormones and increasing feel-good endorphin hormones. But if you exercise and don't eat well, you will feel sluggish and uncomfortable.

• **Tolerance for exercise and recovery** – Again, nutrition is key to sustaining exercise recovery, in fact, nutrition trumps exercise. Eating clean will do amazing things for your stamina and energy, and will aid in allowing the muscle to repair itself as well as engaging muscles that are tired or sore from previous workouts.

• **Fat-loss strategies** – Here's the bad news: as you head farther down the path into menopause, weight gain, and fat-loss patterns shift. And, you guessed it: losing weight becomes harder. Not only that, gaining weight is easier. Women in this stage can pack on five pounds seemingly for no reason.

Hormone shifts play a huge roll in your metabolism. I know, it's not fair, but the good news is that strategies to help are available. Dramatically rotating your carb intake will shock your metabolism. By surprising your body, your metabolism has to respond by adjusting. Carb cycling helps prevent the body from acclimating to a consistent amount of carbs and becoming sluggish.

Chapter 24:
Menopause and Post-Menopause
(45 and older)

• **Hormonal status** – Menopause is the stuff of legends and lore, countless magazine articles, and jokes that your aunts cackled at that you didn't understand when you were a girl.

The trouble with menopause is that many women go into this phase eating the same way they always have, exercising the same way they've always exercised, and going about their daily routines the way they always have. Then they come to me and say, "Oh, I am exhausted, I don't feel right."

Your body is undergoing a massive change, and you need to take this time to get to know it again. This phase of life is so extensive with the amount of recommendations that could be made. Keep in mind this chapter is just scratching the surface.

During this time, your progesterone drops and stays low. Your estrogen goes up-and-down for a while; then plateaus. If a woman has been taking hormone replacement drugs to ease the transition, she typically gives up on it at some point during menopause. It's often an individual decision. To me, hormone replacement therapy seems like it is a way for big business to prey upon women at their most vulnerable point. Most traditional doctors receive very little education on nutrition in medical school, so many resort to hormone replacement as the first line of attack. I disagree with that. I've seen so many symptoms that can be managed through diet and exercise.

- **Nutritional considerations** – A woman going through menopause should still eat for her cycle, even after she no longer has one. Just because you are going through menopause doesn't mean progesterone and estrogen totally shut off. These hormones still cycle through your body, but on a smaller scale than before menopause. You can still take advantage of the benefits of the different stages in the cycle, but be aware that it's not on the same scale as it was. Omega oils can do an excellent job at reducing inflammation.

Most women don't realize they still have a hormonal cycle. My client, Jane, was a funny, sweet lady who worked in a nursing home. Her kids were grown up and gone. She and her husband were enjoying their nearly retired life together taking trips and planning more. She wanted to be able to travel, have lots of energy, and not put on a lot of weight each time she went somewhere. Jane had a goal of losing some weight before her next trip.

She had not had a period in more than 8 years. When I told her that her hormones were still active, she didn't believe me. I had her take and record her basil body temp and send them to me. Low and behold, she had a somewhat regular, 36-day cycle. She was floored. This proved to her that her hormones were still at work in her system.

Now focusing on alternating between warming and cooling foods would be beneficial for her.

She had faster results than I expected. Weight loss was slow and steady, which is good because it leads to permanent change. She experienced an instant change in energy, mental clarity, and steady weight loss. She decided to stay on the hot/cold food cycling while she traveled because it allowed her to continue to feel and look good.

• **Physical and Mental Energy** – Nutrition will have the biggest impact on energy. As the body ages, it needs more to take care of it—more time, energy, focus, and care. It may seem obvious, but people don't realize that as you age, it takes more time and effort to take care of yourself. In your twenties and thirties, you can get away with not taking your vitamins or with eating poorly for a couple of days. But when you are into the menopause phase, not taking care of yourself takes a toll. You have to be more disciplined in your self-care if you want to feel well.

A girlfriend age 36 told me that one night she had friends over. They became so caught up laughing and talking that all they ate was grapes, cheese, and crackers, and they topped it all off with wine. Big mistake. The next day she said she felt like a balloon and worse, saying, "I couldn't get my brain to work."

At age 25, would this have been a problem? Highly unlikely, but for the menopausal women, you don't have that luxury anymore. Remember to take your vitamins, eat well, drink less alcohol, eat less sugar, etc.—or you will certainly feel it!

• **Tolerance for exercise and recovery** – At a minimum, women in this stage should at least walk for exercise. If a woman has never exercised consistently, I recommend walking twenty minutes at least four times a week. Studies have proven that this regimen is beneficial for health, and decreases chances of getting many life-threatening diseases. In addition, women should lift weights at least twice a week to continue maintaining bone strength and density.

• **Fat-loss strategies** – The combination of aging, along with depleted hormones, play a role in making weight loss challenging for most post-menopausal women. Female sex hormone causes fat to be stored in the buttocks, thighs, and hips. When women reach menopause, and the estrogen produced by the ovaries declines, fat migrates from the buttocks, hips, and thighs to the waist. This is why fat acquired later in life is stored in the abdomen. To shed this weight, you have to eat a clean diet and exercise regularly. It may take longer for the scale to move down than it used to, *so don't give up*.

Female Fat Solutions:

1. Each phase of life brings with it the need for changes in nutrition and exercise.

2. Matching nutrition to your phase of life will give you the lasting results you're looking for.

3. Continuing to stay active throughout your lifetime is vital to staying healthy.

Videos:

✓ Estrogen Dominance, Menopause and Nutrition: https://www.youtube.com/watch?v=sut_neJP_tw

Online Resources:

✓ Get on the waitlist for the next 12 Week Menopause Program: www.drbethwestie.com/waitlist

Part 7:

To Summarize

I know sometimes this information can be overwhelming. In the beginning, we talked about the reasons why diet and exercise plans simply don't work for women. I gave you a general idea of how to incorporate specific foods during specific times of your cycle.

If you are looking to implement the information in this book in a way that is custom designed to fit for your body, you're going to want to get on the waitlist for the next 12 Week Program at www.drbethwestie.com/waitlist where you will get a behind-the-scenes look at what the 12 week program entails!

Join the waitlist here: www.drbethwestie.com/waitlist

If you don't want to wait for the next group program to open, and want to work together in a one-to-one capacity, fill out the application at http://bit.ly/DrBethVIP and we will contact you to schedule your FREE one-to-one call with our team to help you determine which program is the right fit, and get you started.

Praise from Those Who Have Used Dr. Westie's Program

"You know that feeling you get when you've met someone whose values align, personality matches, and your business missions are in sync? This is how I felt after meeting and working with Dr. Beth Westie." –Sheila G.

"Going gluten free and sugar free has been easier than I thought, and I feel great. I have more energy, feel less bloated, and my period was much better, which is a big deal. I will keep going and see if I can finally lose some inches, too." Thanks. – Jessica J.

"I, too, have noticed less bloating since going totally gluten free, which is amazing. For me, not having to count calories for every little thing has been liberating. Focusing on the nutrients is so much smarter. Have lost a few pounds and an inch off the waist. Not dramatic but for being pre-menopause, this is very good. Before, I couldn't get any change at all, so I am moving in the right direction now." – Elizabeth N.

"Today I fit into a pair of jeans that had become way to tight. This morning gave them a try and bam...they went on and were not to tight. Felt so good. I am not sure how many pounds I've lost because I have ditched the scale. I have not been feeling like I need a nap in

the afternoon anymore. It still seems strange to eat so much food, but I am getting used to it." — Lindsey S.

"I am a week behind but still down 9 lbs. Many more pounds to lose, but I can feel the difference." – Sarah T.

"I am down 7 pounds so far this month. I have a lot more energy than I had before. Hopefully these results keep coming." – Julie T.

"Losing inches around my hips where I never usually lose." – Melissa V.

"Losing inches around my stomach and thighs." – Kim A.

"I struggle with the scale, and we have a hate/hate relationship. I will wait until the end to weigh myself again, but I know it will be positive results. I have however slept better, have more energy, and realized how awful I felt eating some of the things I did. Low gluten and gluten-free has been awesome for how my body feels." – Molly J.

"Down 6 pounds and several inches since beginning. Definitely feel a difference. So excited for the continued changes." – Kelsey Y.

"I know I'm down inches, down 2 pounds, feel better, sleeping better, eating a ton of food. Keeping on track with each week, and the pores on my face are getting smaller." – Ali R.

"I'm down about 6 pounds and about 8 inches, and my sleep is so much better. It has been a crazy couple of weeks for me with work so I'm struggling and trying to stay the course... "–Heidi S.

"Feeling so good, down 7 pounds, and can only imagine how many inches. My stomach is much flatter and not as bloated.. Followed through with all my cleanse days so far, which in the past had been very hard for me. Can't wait to see what the next 2 weeks brings. And I'm not feeling as awful after I eat meals like I always have, so I think gluten free is for me." – Becky C.

"Does losing weight in your boobs count? No, seriously, it's where I lose first. Workout bra didn't fit yesterday; had to switch to a smaller one." – Victoria G.

"I've lost about 5 pounds and 2 inches off my waist. Truthfully I've stayed on plan about 90% of the time, with some cheating, but overall better and cleaner eating than I've done in over a year. I do keep getting back on track rather than completely fail. That's progress. I'm less puffy and I think the gluten-free foods are helping there." – Megan H.

"I'm loving the food and the options—and who knew coconut oil was so awesome? I also appreciate learning about how my body works and when it needs different things. I love that this plan is adaptable to my life. One of my main "why's" for this program was

to continue to learn about ways I can be healthy and kinder to my body, and I absolutely feel like I'm getting that. Life (and my meal plans) need to be healthy but flexible and sustainable, and this is." – Missy J.

"I lost 7 pounds (I started a little early). After 1 month my cycle lengthened, and I had the longest cycle I've had in two years (27 days). My cycles were 19–21 days with bleeding for 10–12 days. I just started my second cycle on the plan, and it was 25 days. Whoot whoot! I will continue on this plan as I have more to lose. Slow and steady. The warming/cooling is something I'll stick with forever." – Emma R.

"I didn't loose a lot (5 lbs.), but I lost inches and my pants fit better. I now put the scale away for a month. Going to keep following the plan with the hopes that I continue to lose fat and gain muscle." Dr. Beth, thanks for always answering all my crazy questions. – Olivia O.

"Thank you so much. I now see I can get to the person I wanted to be physically. I never thought I would have my life back. " – Sophia F.

"I wanted to let you know that at my gym they tested body fat along with weight and measurements before this challenge. And I know you say the scale isn't a good indicator of success, so I know you would like this. I am down 6% body fat since starting this *program with you. I feel so much better, my clothes fit better, and I finally have the energy I was looking for. You have taught me so much about my body."* THANK YOU. *–Abigail J.*

"I wanted to say thank you. I lost a total of 16 inches in the last 6 weeks. My weight is down 3.7 pounds and my hot flashes are so minimal, it's wonderful. So excited to continue on." Thank you. – Madison S.

"Wanted to share what happened to me this morning. I was running late to my hair appointment because I wanted to make those protein donuts Dr. Beth Westie posted on her website, www.DrBethWestie.com. So being in a hurry, I grabbed a pair of jeans from my closet, hurriedly put them on and thought, thank God they fit without me having to struggle getting into them. While using the bathroom later I noticed the tag inside said size 8 . What? I didn't realize that's what I grabbed. Of course I did a happy dance. So even though the scales hasn't moved a ton, like only 5 pounds, and my measurements are only down a little, things are happening and my clothes are fitting better. So I'll keep plugging away." Thank you. – Hannah G.

"Hi Beth. I wanted to let you know that since I've started your meal plan, I've lost 10.4 pounds. I even had a cheat night of pizza last week, and I've had a few drinks while in the program...plus, this is without working out. Both my hubby and I are loving the meal plan and feel healthier, so thanks. I'm excited about this lifestyle

change. We eat a lot of these foods, but to know when to eat them to work with your body, who knew? I'm so thankful you started this."
– Natalie L.

"I have been doing only the morning routine, and have lost 6 pounds in 3 weeks." –Jill K.

"I had been eating clean and healthy. I was working out 4x/wk. for the last year and a half, and could not drop the last couple pounds I wanted. After starting this plan, I am already down 9 pounds in the first 3 weeks." – Sarah T.

"I have lost over 10 pounds in 4 weeks. I am eating more than I ever have. I have more power and energy for my workouts. I am seeing muscle definition coming so much faster." –Nancy L.

"I had been working out hard for the last 2 years but hadn't been able to break my plateau. Now on this program, in only 4 weeks I am down 15 lbs." – Kathy M.

"I'm only in week 3. I started 5/1, but then my cycle started, so I had to start back at Day 1. Three weeks of chicken/turkey/fish was a bit rough, but really enjoying beef. My hormones are way off; dealt with irregular-to-no cycles for many years, then infertility. Cycles started kind of regulating after I had my kids. I started this knowing it wasn't going to be only a 4-week plan. I honestly thought I wasn't seeing any real change, but then I traveled for work. I followed the *plan as best I could—did the lemon/acv water, used the herbs, packed protein bars, ordered meals/bought meals along the plan as best I could. I knew I was going to be off track, but boy did my body tell me how far off I was. I was crazy bloated, having cravings for sugar and was SO exhausted. I got home, got back on the plan, and it took me through the weekend (4 days), but now I can absolutely tell how I feel different. I have so much energy on this plan that I don't crave anything, not even sweets. I haven't done any measurements, but clothes are fitting better, my workouts are getting easier so I'm able to push myself harder at the gym. It's happening, and now I have to keep with it."* – Samantha E.

"My biggest vice before starting this was sugar, especially a week before my cycle would start. Amazing how eating the right foods eliminated these cravings. Excited to continue this journey and to see how my body starts changing on the outside, too." – Taylor V.

"Isn't it AMAZING...the sugar cravings are gone. And my energy level is better, so I no longer want a nap (even though it is never possible) around 2 in the afternoon." –Jenny A.

******

Hi, I'm Dena S., owner and trainer at UrbanIRON Fitness Studio where we offer small group kettle bell and TRX training. I had been looking for the right model to enhance my nutritional offerings for my clients and knew what I wanted to offer was much more than I had the time to create on my own.

After meeting with Dr. Westie, I knew that her expertise and passion to guide people down the path to improve many areas of their nutrition, was exactly what I had been searching for and jumped into a 6 weekly challenge with my clients.

Dr. Westie's program offered what people needed when they needed it. The knowledge that she shared was extensive, but paced in a way for people to take it in and apply it immediately. Her short/sweet (yet funny) training videos helped to keep people motivated and tweaking things throughout the program.

The list of improvements my clients felt after their 6 weeks on the program impacted them on many levels such as:

- Weight loss (3-20lbs) within the entire group
- Decreased body fat (2-6%)
- Better sleep
- Balanced blood sugar
- Greater mental awareness
- More energy/feeling fueled in workouts

Not everyone experienced the same results; however, everyone experienced results that improved areas of their life that were important for them.

I never question if Dr. Westie's plan is good for my clients — it's whether my clients are ready to work her plan,"

Glossary

Aerobic Training: Aerobic exercise (also known as cardio) is physical exercise of a low-to-high intensity that depends primarily on the aerobic energy-generating process. [xxiii]

Basal Body Temperature: the lowest body temperature attained during rest (usually during sleep). [xxiv]

Body Weight Exercises: These are strength-training exercises that do not require free weights or machines as the individual's own weight provides resistance against gravity. Movements such as the push-up, the pull-up, and the sit-up are some of the most common bodyweight exercises.[xxv]

Clean Diet: A nutrient rich, whole food-based diet plan that does not contain any process or packaged foods.

Fat Soluble: It determines how each vitamin acts within the body. The fat-soluble vitamins are soluble in lipids (fats). These vitamins are usually absorbed in fat globules (called chylomicrons) that travel through the lymphatic system of the small intestines and into the general blood circulation within the body.[xxvi]

Glycogen: A substance that is found in the liver (the organ that cleans the blood) and the muscles, and that stores carbohydrate (a substance that provides energy) and helps to control the level of sugar in the blood[xxvii]

HIIT: High Intensity Interval Training, also called high-intensity intermittent exercise (HIIE) or sprint interval training (SIT), is a form of interval training, a cardiovascular exercise strategy alternating short periods of intense anaerobic exercise with less-intense recovery periods.[xxviii]

Kombucha: is a variety of fermented, lightly effervescent Sweetened black or green tea drinks that are commonly intended as functional beverages for their supposed health benefits.[xxix]

Perimenopause: Perimenopause means "around menopause" and refers to the time during which your body makes the natural transition to menopause, marking the end of the reproductive years.[xxx]

Smooth Muscle: Along with skeletal and cardiac muscle, it is one of the types of muscle tissue in the body. Smooth muscle generally forms the supporting tissue of blood vessels and hollow internal organs, such as the stomach, intestine, and bladder. It is considered smooth because it does not have the microscopic lines (the striations) seen in the other two types of muscle.[xxxi]

Tabata: a form of high-intensity exercise comprising twenty seconds of intense activity followed by ten seconds of rest, conducted over four minutes.[xxxii]

Undenatured: A change in the usual nature of a substance, as by the addition of methanol or acetone to alcohol to render it unfit for drinking, or the change in the physical properties of a substance, such as a protein or nucleic acid, caused by heat or certain chemicals that alter tertiary structure.[xxxiii]

Visceral Fat: Visceral fat is body fat that is stored within the abdominal cavity and is therefore stored around a number of important internal organs such as the liver, pancreas and intestines.[xxxiv]

Endnotes

[i] http://www.scientificamerican.com/article/psychotropic-drugs-affect-men-and-women-differently/

[ii] http://www.slate.com/articles/health_and_science/medical_examiner/2010/07/drug_problem.html

[iii] http://www.palgrave-Journals.com/fr/journal/v72/n1/full/9400055a.html

[iv] http://www.slate.com/articles/health_and_science/medical_examiner/2010/07/drug_problem.html

[v] http://www.scientificamerican.com/article/psychotropic-drugs-affect-men-and-women-differently/

[vi] http://www.medicalnewstoday.com/articles/283808.php

[vii] http://drjamesdobson.org/Solid-Answers/Answers?a=ff773023-2693-410d-b9e1-662f6985be4e

[viii] http://drjamesdobson.org/Solid-Answers/Answers?a=ff773023-2693-410d-b9e1-662f6985be4e

[ix] http://drjamesdobson.org/Solid-Answers/Answers?a=ff773023-2693-410d-b9e1-662f6985be4e

[x] http://www.hindawi.com/journals/jos/2011/702735/

[xi] http://www.naturalnews.com/042753_Epsom_salt_baths_remarkable_health_benefits_detoxificatin_technique.html#ixzz3VEZQ646y

[xii] https://www.vitamindcouncil.org/health-conditions/cognitive-impairment

[xiii] http://sleepfoundation.org/sleep-topics/women-and-sleep

[xiv] http://sleepfoundation.org/sleep-topics/women-and-sleep

[xv] http://aje.oxfordjournals.org/content/early/2013/01/15/aje.kws422.full

[xvi] http://sleepfoundation.org/sleep-topics/women-and-sleep

[xvii] http://psychology.about.com/od/statesofconsciousness/a/SleepStages.htm.

[xviii] http://www.pewsocialtrends.org/2013/03/14/modern-parenthood-roles-of-moms-and-dads-converge-as-they-balance-work-and-family/)

[xix] http://www.forbes.com/sites/heidigranthalvorson/2012/12/23/nine-ways-successful-people-defeat-stress/

[xx] http://www.womenshealthmag.com/health/side-effects-of-stress

[xxi] http://www.academia.edu/350423/The_effects_of_stress_on_food_choice_mood_and_bodyweight_in_healthy_women
[xxii] https://circle.ubc.ca/handle/2429/7306
[xxiii] https://en.wikipedia.org/wiki/Aerobic_exercise
[xxiv] https://en.wikipedia.org/wiki/Basal_body_temperature
[xxv] https://en.wikipedia.org/wiki/Bodyweight_exercise
[xxvi] http://www.medicinenet.com/script/main/art.asp?articlekey=10736
[xxvii] http://dictionary.cambridge.org/us/dictionary/english/glycogen
[xxviii] https://en.wikipedia.org/wiki/High-intensity_interval_training
[xxix] https://en.wikipedia.org/wiki/Kombucha
[xxx] http://www.mayoclinic.org/diseases-conditions/perimenopause/home/ovc-20253772
[xxxi] http://www.medicinenet.com/script/main/art.asp?articlekey=5514
[xxxii] https://www.collinsdictionary.com/us/submission/12836/Tabata
[xxxiii] http://medical-dictionary.thefreedictionary.com/Undenatured
[xxxiv] http://www.diabetes.co.uk/body/visceral-fat.html

Made in the USA
Columbia, SC
14 October 2021